Laboratory Activity Guide for

Anatomy & Physiology

Brian H. Kipp

Department of Biomedical Sciences
Grand Valley State University
Allendale, Michigan

Wolters Kluwer Health | Lippincott Williams & Wilkins

Philadelphia · Baltimore · New York · London
Buenos Aires · Hong Kong · Sydney · Tokyo

Executive Editor: David Troy
Associate Product Manager: Erin M. Cosyn
Marketing Manager: Shauna Kelley
Product Director: Eric Branger
Compositor: Aptara, Inc.
Designer: Larry Didona

© 2012 by LIPPINCOTT WILLIAMS & WILKINS, a WOLTERS KLUWER business

351 West Camden Street   Two Commerce Square
Baltimore, Maryland 21201   2001 Market Street
                                            Philadelphia, Pennsylvania 19103

Printed in China

All rights reserved. This book is protected by copyright. No part of this book may be reproduced or transmitted in any form or by any means, including as photocopies or scanned-in or other electronic copies, or utilized by any information storage and retrieval system without written permission from the copyright owner, except for brief quotations embodied in critical articles and reviews. Materials appearing in this book prepared by individuals as part of their official duties as U.S. government employees are not covered by the above-mentioned copyright. To request permission, please contact Lippincott Williams & Wilkins at Two Commerce Square, 2001 Market Street, Philadelphia, PA 19103, via email at permissions@lww.com, or via website at lww.com (products and services).

9 8 7 6 5 4 3 2 1

Library of Congress Cataloging-in-Publication

CIP data available on request.

DISCLAIMER

Care has been taken to confirm the accuracy of the information present and to describe generally accepted practices. However, the authors, editors, and publisher are not responsible for errors or omissions or for any consequences from application of the information in this book and make no warranty, expressed or implied, with respect to the currency, completeness, or accuracy of the contents of the publication. Application of this information in a particular situation remains the professional responsibility of the practitioner; the clinical treatments described and recommended may not be considered absolute and universal recommendations.

The authors, editors, and publisher have exerted every effort to ensure that drug selection and dosage set forth in this text are in accordance with the current recommendations and practice at the time of publication. However, in view of ongoing research, changes in government regulations, and the constant flow of information relating to drug therapy and drug reactions, the reader is urged to check the package insert for each drug for any change in indications and dosage and for added warnings and precautions. This is particularly important when the recommended agent is a new or infrequently employed drug.

Some drugs and medical devices presented in this publication have Food and Drug Administration (FDA) clearance for limited use in restricted research settings. It is the responsibility of the health care providers to ascertain the FDA status of each drug or device planned for use in their clinical practice.

To purchase additional copies of this book, call our customer service department at **(800) 638-3030** or fax orders to **(301) 223-2320**. International customers should call **(301) 223-2300**.

Visit Lippincott Williams & Wilkins on the Internet: http://www.lww.com. Lippincott Williams & Wilkins customer service representatives are available from 8:30 am to 6:00 pm, EST.

This laboratory manual is dedicated to my beautiful wife Nicole and my great kids, Caleb, Ethan and Abby. Without their support and patience, this would not be possible.

Thank you to John Capodilupo for all the help teaching and designing courses.

Thomas Bukoskey, DPT
Assistant Professor
Tennessee State University
Nashville, TN

Luciano Debeljuk, PhD, MD
Associate Professor
Southern Illinois University
Carbondale, IL

Mandi Dupain, PhD
Assistant Professor
Millersville University
Millersville, PA

Chaya Gopalan, PhD
Professor
St. Louis Community College
Ferguson, MO

Ana Hayes-Perez, PhD, MD
Assistant Professor
Tennessee State University
Nashville, TN

Mary Puglia, PhD
Professor
Central Arizona College
Apache Junction, AZ

Sanda Stewart, MS
Professor
Vincennes University
Vincennes, IN

Teresa Trendler, MS
Professor
Pasadena City College
Pasadena, CA

Why another Anatomy and Physiology laboratory manual? There are literally hundreds of A&P lab manuals in the marketplace today, so why did I see the need to create yet another one? My reasoning: simplicity, clarity, and cost effective for both students and schools. I set out to create a lab manual that presented anatomy and physiology in a simple and easily understandable way. This manual functions as a workbook to effectively guide students through any introductory anatomy and physiology course. It is designed to complement any instructor's lecture material as well as any basic anatomy and physiology textbook. It complements the partner book without competing for the student's attention. Rather, students can use the lab manual to work with the book, not separately from the book.

In an attempt to be a one-size-fits-all, many manuals will contain not only anatomy and physiology, but also pathophysiology and pharmacology. As a result students who are trying to learn basic A&P struggle with the pathophysiology and pharmacology information much too early in their career. This distracts students from the topic at hand and can prevent them from developing a foundation in the basic science that is necessary for future success. Here I present the anatomy and physiology that all health students must know. Once students master the material presented in a laboratory section, they will have a firm foundation and will be well prepared to progress in their studies.

Too often lab manuals reproduce material that is already presented in the lecture and textbook. Students are often overwhelmed with the amount of information and are unsure of what they truly need to know. In this manual I have streamlined and simplified the presentation of the material to be at the appropriate level for introductory health students. This simple, straightforward delivery covers all the basic information, and leaves room for instructors to add any examples they choose. Every organ system is presented with an emphasis on the relevant anatomy and physiology. Simple experiments are proposed that clearly demonstrate complex topics. Through figure labeling and answering questions based on function, students are able to make connections between form and function, without being overwhelmed with unnecessarily complex concepts that are beyond what the introductory health student needs to know. Rather than provide complicated experiments that require costly equipment that many labs may not have, I present simple activities that rely on basic equipment available in almost all lab settings to enforce the critical content needed at the introductory level.

In my 10 years as an instructor I have found lab activities like those included here to be effective learning tools for my students. The hands-on approach and tangible learning process of lab activities reinforce the material in a way that is not possible with lectures and reading alone, yet the simplicity of these activities focuses on the core anatomy and physiology material without overwhelming the student with extras, the way many other lab manuals do. I hope you and your students will find this lab manual to be as beneficial as my students and I have.

Brian H. Kipp

CONTENTS

General Laboratory Safety

Objectives

After completing this laboratory exercise, students will be able to:

1. Review basic safety procedures for the laboratory.
2. Be aware of potential hazards in the laboratory.

Overview

During this semester's lab course you may encounter some potentially dangerous materials or situations. In this short overview we will review how you should conduct yourself in the laboratory to minimize these situations and what to do in the event of an emergency.

Exercise

Exercise 1.1: Basic safety practices of the laboratory

Estimated lab time: 30 minutes

Exercise 1.1

Basic Safety Practices of the Laboratory

The potential hazards you may encounter in the laboratory include sharp objects (scalpel, broken glass), fluids (perhaps urine or blood), and basic day-to-day hazards. Most days, there will be nothing to worry about, but it is good practice to always be prepared. Some of the practices that will ensure you and your classmates' safety are:

1. Do not eat or drink in the laboratory!

2. Locate the emergency exits for the lab.

3. Locate the fire extinguisher and fire alarm panel in the lab.

4. Know where the first aid kit is kept.

5. Always wear old clothes to the lab.

6. Make sure you have closed-toed shoes in the lab to protect your feet from dropped materials.

7. Put all glass and biowaste in the proper containers as directed by your instructor.

8. Notify your instructor of any spills or broken equipment immediately.

9. Decontaminate and clean all surfaces when you are finished with the exercise of the day.

10. Notify your instructor if you have any medical conditions that may be of concern.

11. Keep all equipment and models away from the edge of the table.

12. When appropriate, wear eye protection.

13. When appropriate, wear protective clothing such as a lab coat and keep all long hair tied back.

Study Questions

Answer the following questions as completely as possible.

1. Why do you think it is inappropriate to eat in the lab?

   _____

   _____

   _____

2. What is the first thing you should do when a spill occurs in the lab?

   _____

   _____

   _____

3. What safety equipment would be appropriate when boiling a solution for a laboratory exercise?

   _____

   _____

   _____

4. When a glass beaker is broken in the lab, where should you dispose of the glass?

   _____

   _____

   _____

5. A female student has just found out she is pregnant. Should she quit the lab? If not, what course of action should she follow and why?

   _____

   _____

   _____

Introduction to Human Anatomy

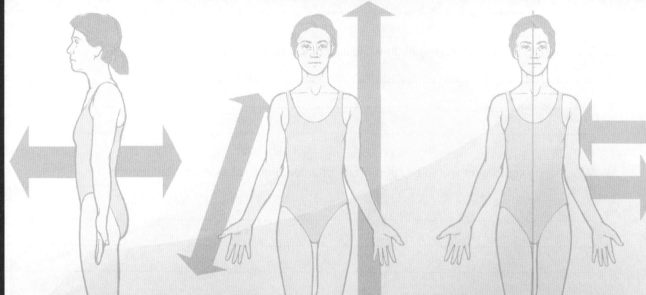

Objectives

After completing this laboratory exercise, students will be able to:

1. Define and locate an example of each of the major anatomical terms.
2. Determine and demonstrate anatomical directions.
3. Determine and locate anatomical cavities.
4. Locate and describe anatomical planes and sections.

Overview

To fully describe anatomical structures we need to have points of reference. This laboratory exercise will introduce you to many of the directional and commonly used descriptive terms in anatomy. Use your textbook, the models provided, your lab partners, and your own body to become familiar with the use of these terms. It is important that you are comfortable with

them, as you will need to use them regularly throughout your Anatomy & Physiology course and continuing on into your healthcare career.

Lab Materials

It is useful to have a wide variety of models available to demonstrate the different directions, planes, and cavities.

■ Human torso models
■ Organ models
■ Bone models

Exercises

Exercise 2.1: Use of anatomical directional terms
Exercise 2.2: Anatomical planes and sections
Exercise 2.3: Body cavities

Estimated Lab time: 60 minutes

Use of Anatomical Directional Terms

Refer to your textbook to perform the following exercises.

1. Define/describe the terms in the table and provide a short description or example of the term.

Term	Region/Reference	Example
Anterior		
Ventral		
Posterior		
Cranial		
Superior		
Caudal		
Inferior		
Medial		
Lateral		
Proximal		
Distal		
Superficial		
Deep		

2. Locate an example of each term in the table using the available models and indicate on Figures 2.1 and 2.2 where these regions are located.

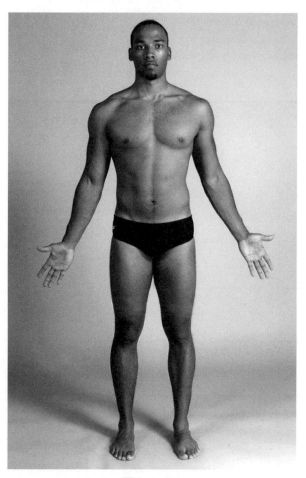

Figure 2.1

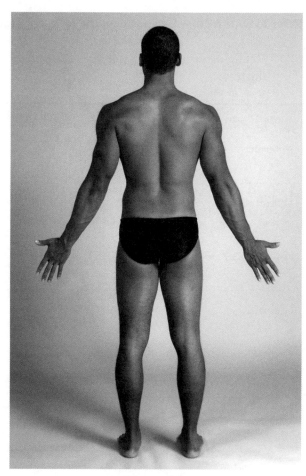

Figure 2.2

3. Locate and label the following anatomical directions on Figure 2.3:

- Cranial
- Caudal
- Posterior
- Anterior
- Superior
- Inferior

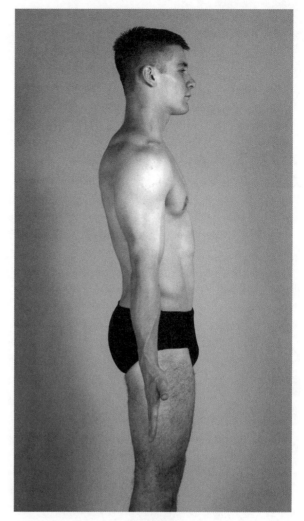

Figure 2.3

4. Using one of the models provided in the lab, identify the same six directions. Then locate them on your lab partner.

5. Locate and label the following anatomical directions on Figure 2.4:

- Lateral
- Medial
- Proximal
- Distal

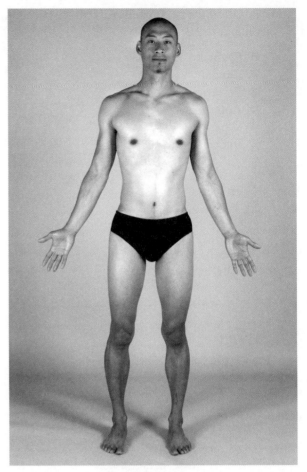

Figure 2.4

6. Using one of the models provided in the lab, identify the same four directions. Then locate them on your lab partner.

Anatomical Planes and Sections

Label the following planes and sections in Figure 2.5:

- ▣ Transverse plane
  - ☐ Superior section
  - ☐ Inferior section
- ▣ Frontal plane
  - ☐ Anterior section
  - ☐ Posterior section
- ▣ Sagittal plane
  - ☐ Left section
  - ☐ Right section

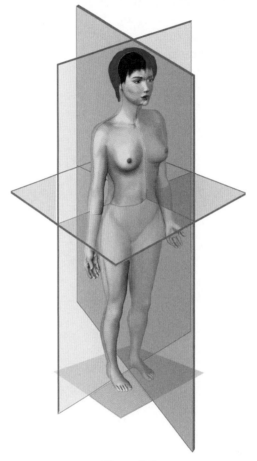

Figure 2.5

Body Cavities

Exercise 2.3

Label the following body cavities in Figure 2.6:

- Thoracic cavity
- Spinal canal
- Abdominopelvic cavity
    - ☐ Pelvic cavity
    - ☐ Abdominal cavity

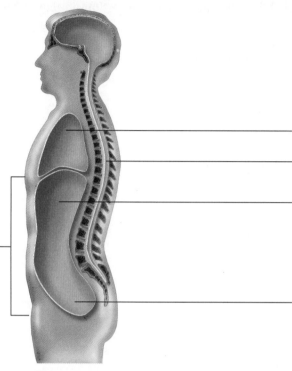

Figure 2.6

Study Questions

1. Your hand is _____ to your elbow.

2. Your brain is located with the _____ cavity.

3. Your foot is _____ to your pelvis.

4. The skin is _____ to underlying structures.

5. Your navel is on the _____ axis whereas your arms are _____ to the longitudinal axis.

6. The lungs are found within the _____ cavity.

7. The heart is found within the _____ cavity.

8. Your face is on the _____ of the body.

9. Your shoulder is _____ in relation to your hand, which is _____ to your shoulder.

10. The _____ plane is parallel to the long axis of the body.

Cellular Anatomy and the Microscope

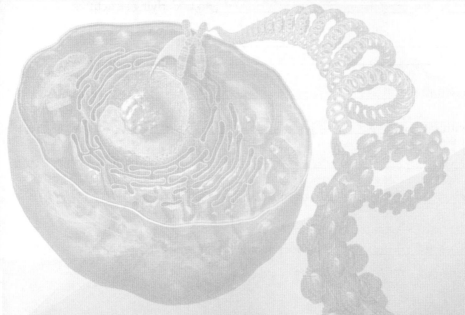

Objectives

After completing this laboratory exercise, students will be able to:

1. Name and identify the major parts of the microscope.
2. Identify the organelles of a typical human cell.
3. Define/describe the function of each organelle.
4. Describe the stages of mitosis.

Overview

In order to understand anatomy and physiology, one must have an understanding of the fundamental units of life, cells. This laboratory exercise is intended as a review of basic cellular anatomy and physiology and will acquaint you with the microscope and its operation.

Lab Materials

- Microscope
- Lens paper
- Letter "e" mounted on microscope slide
- Animal cell model
- Toothpicks
- Glass slides and cover slips
- Iodine
- Animal cell mitosis stage slides

Exercises

Exercise 3.1: Observations with a microscope
Exercise 3.2: Typical human cell and organelles
Exercise 3.3: Mitosis and cellular division

Estimated lab time: 90 minutes

USE OF THE MICROSCOPE

The following provides a quick overview of microscope use for the student unfamiliar with binocular microscopes. This section will also review terminology and procedures for operating mechanical stage microscopes. Review this before each laboratory session utilizing microscopes.

Some Basic Techniques

1. Use lens paper to clean the lenses on the eyepieces and the objectives. Do not use Kimwipes or paper towel due to their ability to scratch glass.

2. Remember to adjust light for the best possible view of the field. Light adjustment can be achieved in two ways:
   (a) Adjusting the iris diaphragm on the substage condenser.
   (b) Raising or lowering the substage condenser.

3. On some microscopes, or on the transformers used with some models, there is a rheostat that can be used to vary the intensity of the light source.

4. Light should be increased upon switching to a higher level of magnification, and decreased when switching to a lower magnification.

5. Begin focusing with the 10× objective. Use the coarse adjustment knob to bring the field into focus. Sharpen the focus with the fine adjustment knob.

6. To use a higher level of magnification, swing the objective from the 10× to the 40× ("high dry"). The lenses should be sufficiently parfocal so that a little turning of the fine adjustment knob will bring the field of view into focus. Do not use the coarse adjustment knob at the higher levels of magnification, as it is far too easy to break a slide or damage an objective lens. ***Remember to adjust the light when changing the magnification.***

Total Magnification

To figure the total magnification of an image that you are viewing through a microscope, take the power of the objective lens and multiply that by the power of the eyepiece lenses. So, if you are using the 10× objective lens and the eyepiece has a magnification of 10× also, the total magnification would be $10 \times 10 = 100$.

Use of Binocular Eyepieces

The two eyepieces are mounted to permit moving them closer together or farther apart to match the distance between the eyes of the user. As you look through the two eyepieces, adjust the distance between them until the two fields merge. Binocular viewing is much easier on the eyes than monocular work.

Use of the Mechanical Stage

Microscopes used in introductory courses usually have clips to hold the slide in place, and the person moves the slide back and forth to examine different parts of the slide. With the mechanical stage, a hinged spring clamp holds the slide in place, and one moves the slide in its slide holder by turning the knobs. One knob moves the slide holder in the left and right direction, the other in the forward and backward direction. There are two scales, which can be read if you want to record the location of an object on a prepared slide so that it can be found upon subsequent viewings.

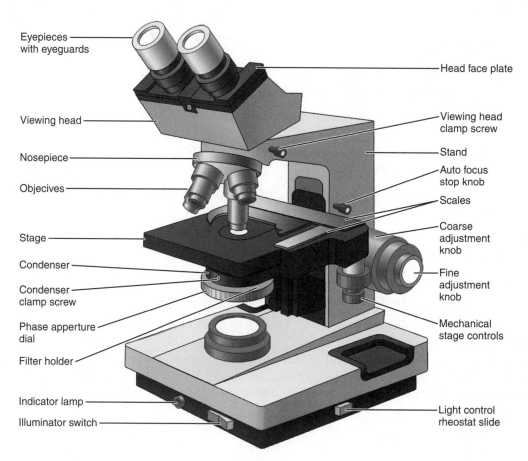

Figure 3.1

Observations with a Microscope

1. Obtain a prepared slide of the letter "e." Place the slide on the stage and secure it so that it will not slip. Turn on the light source and place the low power lens in the viewing position.

2. Using the coarse adjustment knob, bring the stage as close to the low power lens as you can. Now, slowly turn the coarse adjustment knob until you can see the letter "e". Use the fine focus to bring the letter into sharp focus.

3. Once the letter is clearly visible, rotate the nosepiece to the next higher objective lens. The image should be in focus, but if it is not, use the fine focus. **NEVER USE THE COARSE ADJUSTMENT ON HIGHER POWER LENSES,** it may cause the slide to crash into the lens, damaging both the lens and the slide.

4. As you increase the magnification, you may need to adjust the intensity of the light. Depending on your microscope, you may have a slider (as in Figure 3.1) or a diaphragm under the stage.

Typical Human Cell and Organelles

The typical human cell contains many important organelles and structures. Using your textbook, provide a brief explanation of the function of each organelle/structure. Be sure to include in your description the important elements shown in each figure.

1. Plasma membrane

   Description of function:

   _____

   _____

   _____

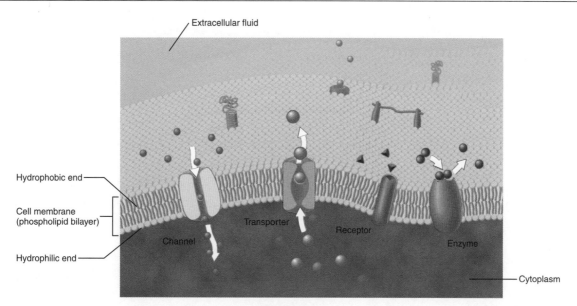

Figure 3.2

2. Nucleus and nucleolus

Description of function:

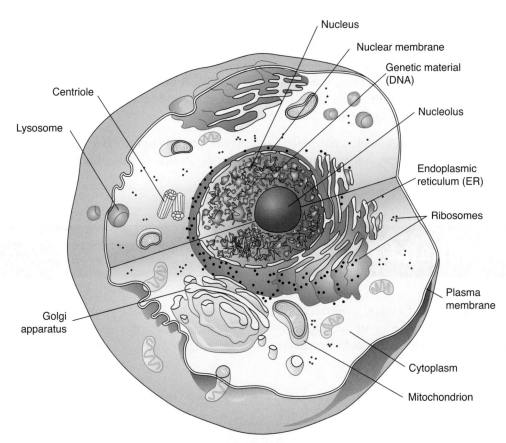

Figure 3.3

3. Mitochondria

Description of function:

_____

_____

_____

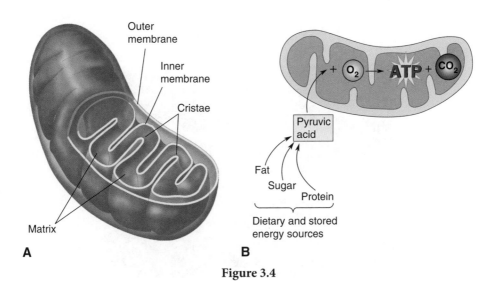

Figure 3.4

4. Endoplasmic reticulum and ribosomes

Description of function:

_____

_____

_____

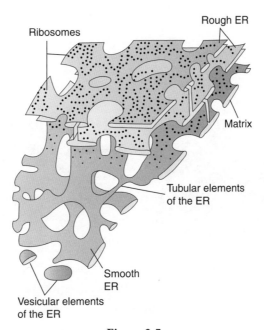

Figure 3.5

5. Golgi apparatus

Description of function:

_____

_____

_____

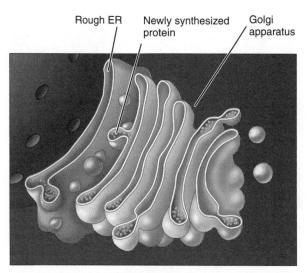

Figure 3.6

6. Lysosomes (figure depicts lysosome in action in a white blood cell)

Description of function:

_____

_____

_____

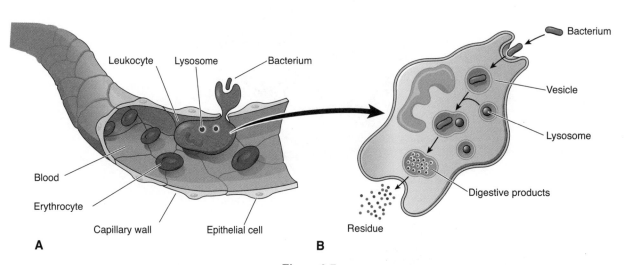

Figure 3.7

7. Centrioles

Description of function:

_____

_____

_____

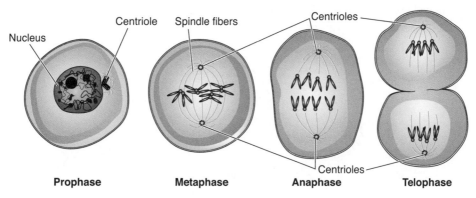

Figure 3.8

8. Cytoplasm

Description of function:

_____

_____

_____

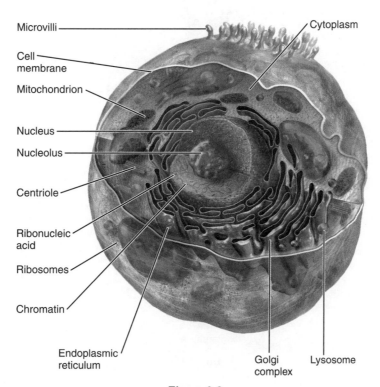

Figure 3.9

Mitosis and Cellular Division

The cell cycle describes the life cycle of each individual cell. As an organism grows, cells divide and tissues enlarge. Once the organism reaches maturity, most cells enter a phase of maturity and stasis, known as G0, but some cell types continue to divide. Figure 3.10 illustrates the different phases of the cell cycle, and particularly the phases of mitosis.

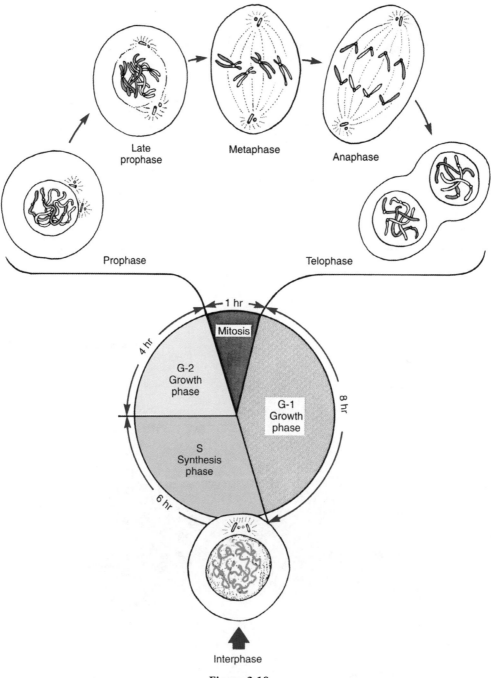

Figure 3.10

1. Describe the purpose of G1, S, G2, and Mitosis.

_____

_____

_____

_____

_____

Instructions:

Obtain a set of mitosis slides from your lab instructor and observe each stage. Then draw the chromosomal arrangement/state during each phase and provide a brief description of each stage:

1. Prophase

Description:

_____

_____

_____

2. Late prophase

Description:

_____

_____

_____

3. Metaphase

Description:

_____

_____

_____

4. Anaphase

Description:

_____

_____

_____

5. Telophase

Description:

_____

_____

_____

Study Questions

Instructions:

1. Write the name of the indicated microscope component on the lines below.

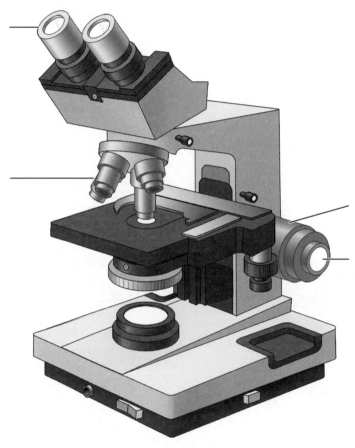

Figure 3.11

2. When looking at a slide depicting prophase, your objective is set at 40× and the eye piece is 12.5×. What is the total magnification of the image?

   _____

   _____

   _____

3. Which organelle is responsible for protein assembly?

   _____

   _____

   _____

4. Where in the cell is genetic material stored?

_____

_____

_____

5. Which organelle is responsible for the breakdown of foreign or dead material in the cell?

_____

_____

_____

6. Which organelle is responsible for modifying proteins?

_____

_____

_____

7. In which phase of the cell cycle does DNA replication occur?

_____

_____

_____

8. In which phase of the cell cycle are the chromosomes dispersed? When do they condense?

_____

_____

_____

9. _____ is the phase where the chromosomes begin moving toward the centrioles.

10. In which phase do mature adult cells spend most of their time?

_____

_____

_____

11. In metaphase, the chromosomes are _____.

Osmosis and Diffusion

Objectives

After completing this laboratory exercise, students will be able to:

1. Define diffusion.
2. Explain the physiological process of diffusion.
3. Define osmosis.
4. Explain the physiological process of osmosis.
5. Apply the concept of osmosis and diffusion to the human body.

Overview

Osmosis and diffusion are the basic processes of cellular transport. The movement of solutes and fluids drives many of the cell's basic functions. In this lab you will become familiar with these fundamental concepts.

Terms and Definitions

isotonic: A solution that has the same salt concentration as the normal cells of the body and blood.

hypertonic: A solution that has a higher salt concentration than the normal cells of the body and blood.

hypotonic: A solution that has less salt concentration than the normal cells of the body and blood.

osmolarity: The concentration of all solute particles dissolved in a solution.

osmosis: The movement of water across a semipermeable membrane from an area of low concentration of nonpenetrating particles to an area of high concentration of nonpenetrating particles.

tonicity: The nature of a solute that either prevents or promotes osmosis from occurring.

Lab Materials

- Ink or dark stain
- Three small beakers
- Ice
- Hot plate
- Dropper
- Thermometer
- Stopwatch
- Test tubes
- Ruler

- Isotonic saline 0.85% NaCl
- Hypertonic saline 3.0% NaCl
- Hypotonic saline 0.2% NaCl
- Sheep or human blood

Exercises

Exercise 4.1: Simple diffusion
Exercise 4.2: Osmosis

Estimated lab time: 60 minutes

Simple Diffusion

Diffusion is the process by which molecules intermingle as a result of their kinetic energy of random motion resulting in the passive movement of a solute from an area of greater concentration to an area of lower concentration. **Osmosis** is the movement of water from an area of higher concentration to an area of lower concentration across the semipermeable membrane. Neither process depends on energy generated by living organisms, thus they are referred to as passive processes.

For diffusion to take place there must be a concentration gradient of a solute. The rate of diffusion is dependent on factors such as temperature, particle size, and the concentration gradient. A concentration gradient is the difference in concentration of the substance in question between two locations.

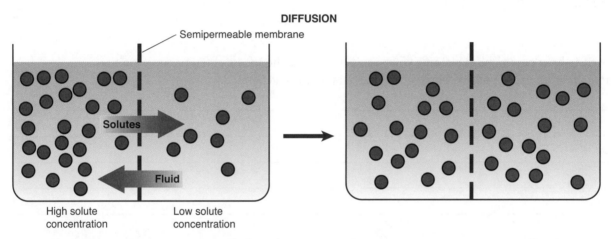

DIFFUSION

Semipermeable membrane

Solutes

Fluid

High solute concentration

Low solute concentration

Figure 4.1 Diffusion: movement of solutes from an area of greater concentration to an area of lesser concentration, leading ultimately to equalization of the solute concentrations.

Instructions:

1. Obtain a clean beaker and place it on top of a white sheet of paper.

2. Fill the beaker half full with room temperature water.

3. Put two drops of stain into the beaker and measure the time it takes for full diffusion to occur.

4. Repeat the experiment with cold and hot water and record the time below.

Room Temperature _____ °C   Time: _____ seconds

Cold Temperature _____ °C   Time: _____ seconds

Warm Temperature _____ °C   Time: _____ seconds

Study Questions

1. Write a brief paragraph explaining your results regarding the effects of temperature on the rate of diffusion. In your explanation use the data that you generated.

   _____

   _____

   _____

   _____

   _____

2. Define the following:

   a. Diffusion

   _____

   _____

   b. Solute

   _____

   _____

   c. Solvent

   _____

   _____

3. Provide an example in the human body where diffusion takes place.

   _____

   _____

   _____

Osmosis

Water is essentially the only molecule that moves freely between cells and the extracellular fluid. It moves between cells and through cells in response to solutes in solution. These solutes are either penetrating or nonpenetrating to the cell membrane. The movement of water is termed osmosis. **Osmosis** is the movement of water across a semipermeable membrane from an area of low concentration of nonpenetrating particles to an area of high concentration of nonpenetrating particles. As a rule, water moves to dilute the area of more concentrated solute.

OSMOSIS

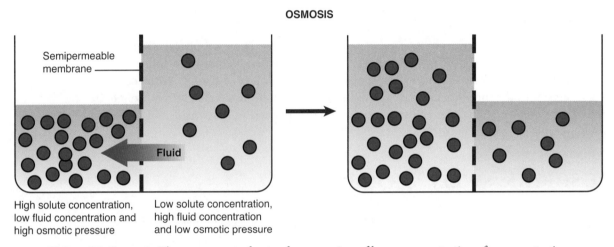

High solute concentration, low fluid concentration and high osmotic pressure

Low solute concentration, high fluid concentration and low osmotic pressure

Figure 4.2 Osmosis: The movement of water from a region of lesser concentration of nonpenetrating particles toward an area of higher concentration of nonpenetrating particles.

In order to maintain cellular integrity outside of the body, cells must be placed in an isotonic solution. The unique characteristics of isotonic solutions prevent water from entering or leaving the cell. As a result, cells placed in an isotonic solution neither shrink nor swell. In this experiment we will be using red blood cells (RBCs) to determine the **tonicity** of the solution.

One way of testing tonicity is to observe the microscopic effect a solution has on RBCs. Since an effectively nonpenetrating solute does not change the **osmolarity** of the cell, water movement is regulated entirely by the osmolarity of the solution. The concentration of the solute determines the direction of water movement. An isosmotic (equal concentration of particles in ICF and ECF) solution made of a nonpenetrating solute causes no visible change, this solution is called an **isotonic** solution.

If cells are placed in a hyperosmotic solution (greater concentration in ECF than ICF) made of a nonpenetrating solute, water leaves the cell until solute concentration inside the cell is equal to the solute concentration of the surrounding media. The cell becomes crenated, with a prickly appearance. Since this solution causes water to move out of the cell, it is called a **hypertonic** solution.

If cells are placed in a hypo-osmotic solution, using an effectively nonpenetrating solute, water enters the cell until the solute concentration inside the cell equals the solute concentration outside the cell. The movement of water into the cell causes swelling. As the cell swells the membrane stretches to the point of bursting, eventually lysing the cell. In RBCs this process is known as hemolysis. Because the solution causes water to move into the cell, it is called a **hypotonic** solution.

Generally, the more hypertonic the solution, the more rapid the crenation will occur. Conversely, the more hypotonic the solution, the more rapid the cell will undergo hemolysis. This depends on the nature of the solute particle remaining essentially nonpenetrating.

OSMOTIC HEMOLYSIS AS A TEST FOR MEMBRANE PERMEABILITY

It is nearly impossible to create an isotonic solution with a solute that penetrates cell membranes. The rate of hemolysis is greatly dependent on the speed at which the solute penetrates the cell membrane. Lipid solubility, molecular size, and ionic charges all contribute to the speed at which a solute penetrates the cell membrane. Cells placed in a solution with a quickly penetrating solute hemolyze rapidly; slower penetrating solutes cause more gradual hemolysis. It is possible, then, to use hemolysis as a means of measuring the membrane permeability rate for different solutes.

In the lab, membrane permeability can be measured through the visual observation of blood suspensions. By timing the rate of osmotic hemolysis the permeability of a solute can be assessed. A nonhemolyzed erythrocyte suspension appears cloudy or turbid. As the cells undergo hemolysis, the turbidity decreases until the suspension becomes clear, even though the red or pink color remains. Generally, hemolysis occurs quickest in suspensions of solutes with high membrane permeabilities.

THE SHRINK, SWELL, OR POP TEST

Instructions: Students will conduct observations of hemolysis, swelling, and crenation to determine the tonicity of a solution.

All students must wear protective gloves when working with blood. Even though the sample of blood used is guaranteed to be HIV negative, you should always practice universal precautions. Is important to treat all blood solutions in the 10% bleached solution before discarding the solution. Do not dispose blood solutions directly into glass waste containers.

Preparing Stock Blood Suspension

Obtain a glass test tube and fill 2/3 of the tube with isotonic saline. Your lab instructor will add enough blood to your tube of saline to make it a rich red color. This blood suspension will be used in the following studies and experiments as your stock solution. Before each use, mix the blood solution by placing a small piece of film over the top of the tube and slowly invert the tube 4–5 times being very careful not to make bubbles.

Studies with the Microscope

A. Observe a prepared blood smear

1. Determine which side of the slide has the smear of blood (it will appear dull) and be sure that side is up when placing the slide on the microscope stage.

2. Begin with the 10× objective and find a field near the edge of the smear where the cells are scattered rather than matted together. The cells will appear as small grains.

3. Now switch to the 40× objective lens. The vast majority of the cells will be erythrocytes (RBCs): biconcave disks with no nuclei. The other cells you may see are white blood cells (leukocytes) and will differ in that they are larger and have a purple stained nucleus.

B. Prepare a wet mount slide of normal RBCs

1. Obtain a clean dry slide and cover slip, being careful to only touch the cover slip on the edge.

2. Apply small "drops" of Vaseline to two corners of the cover slip (on the same side).

3. Take a drop of the stock blood solution you prepared earlier and place it on the slide.

4. Drag the edge of the cover slip that does not have Vaseline until it makes contact with the drop of blood.

5. Once the cover slip has made contact with the blood drop the Vaseline treated side gently down on top of the drop of blood.

6. Examine the slide under the microscope, starting with the lowest objective. Focus on the RBCs (the small grains again).

7. Move to the next highest objective lens and observe the cells. When moving to higher objective lenses be careful not to allow the lens to hit the slide. You should be able to see biconcave disks.

C. Observe cells in solutions of different solute concentrations

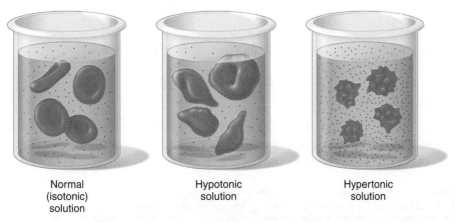

Normal
(isotonic)
solution

Hypotonic
solution

Hypertonic
solution

Figure 4.3 Effects of osmosis on red blood cells in different concentrations: isotonic, hypotonic, and hypertonic solutions.

1. Obtain three test tubes and label them A, B, and C. Mark off 1.5 cm from the bottom.

2. Fill tube A to the 1.5 cm mark with 3.0% NaCl, tube B with 0.85% NaCl, and tube C with 0.2% NaCl solution.

3. Add a squirt (pipette tip filled to where the diameter widens to maximal width) of your stock RBC suspension to each tube and gently mix.

4. Prepare a wet mount (slide) of each newly made suspension from tubes A, B, and C. Examine each slide under the microscope and compare the cells' shape to Figure 4.3 and record your observations in the table below.
   - Under "Appearance of Cells" list as normal, crenated, swollen, or absent according to what you see.
   - Under "Tonicity of Solution" list the appropriate prefix hyper-, iso-, or hypo-, according to what happened to the majority of cells

Observations of Blood Cells in NaCl Solutions of Various Concentrations			
NaCl Conc.	**Appearance of Cells**	**Tonicity of Solution**	**Solution Appearance**
3.0%			
0.85%			
0.20%			

D. Observe hemolysis

When blood cells from your suspension are added to a clear isotonic solution, the solution becomes turbid. If cells are added to a hypotonic solution, hemolysis occurs and the solution turns clear.

1. Examine your three test tubes from part C. Are any of the tubes clear? If you have difficulty telling, hold each solution in front of your lab manual and see if you can read the letters clearly. If the letters appear clear, then the cells have hemolyzed. If the letters are at all cloudy or fuzzy then the cells have not.

2. Repeat the procedure from part C, but substitute the unknown solutions labeled A, B, and C from your instructor. Do not make wet mounts; rather just observe the change in turbidity, and use these observations to determine the tonicity of each solution.

Observations of Blood Cells in Unknown Solutions of Various Concentrations		
Unknown Solution	**Solution Appearance**	**Tonicity of Solution**
A		
B		
C		

Study Questions

1. Define osmosis.

_____

_____

_____

2. Define the following:

   a. Isotonic solution

   _____

   _____

   b. Hypertonic solution

   _____

   _____

   c. Hypotonic solution

   _____

   _____

   d. Tonicity

   _____

   _____

   e. Hemolysis

   _____

   _____

   f. Crenate

   _____

   _____

3. What caused the crenation of blood cells in this laboratory exercise?

   _____

   _____

   _____

4. What caused the hemolysis of the cells in this laboratory exercise?

_____

_____

_____

5. How is osmosis relevant to administration of intravenous fluids?

_____

_____

_____

Basic Histology

Objectives

After completing this laboratory exercise, students will be able to:

1. Name the four basic tissues of the human body.
2. Observe and identify a variety of prepared tissue sections with a microscope.
3. Provide an example of where each tissue studied in this laboratory may be found in the body.
4. Provide the basic function of each identified tissue/cell type.

Overview

To understand physiology, one must first possess an understanding of anatomy. In human beings, form and function are closely related. This laboratory exercise is intended as a review of basic cellular anatomy (histology) and will acquaint you with the microscope and its operation.

Lab Materials

- Microscope
- Complete set of tissue slides including epithelial, connective, muscle, and nervous tissues.
- Lens paper

Exercises

Exercise 5.1: Simple squamous epithelium
Exercise 5.2: Stratified squamous epithelium
Exercise 5.3: Simple cuboidal epithelium
Exercise 5.4: Simple columnar epithelium
Exercise 5.5: Pseudostratified ciliated columnar epithelium
Exercise 5.6: Transitional epithelium
Exercise 5.7: Dense regular connective tissue
Exercise 5.8: Dense irregular connective tissue
Exercise 5.9: Hyaline cartilage
Exercise 5.10: Elastic cartilage
Exercise 5.11: Bone (osseous tissue)
Exercise 5.12: Skeletal muscle
Exercise 5.13: Cardiac muscle
Exercise 5.14: Smooth muscle
Exercise 5.15: Neural tissue

Estimated lab time: 90 minutes

Instructions:

This lab is set up with a number of different exercise stations, each with a type of tissue to be examined. At each station, you will find a microscope and histological sections already placed under the objective lens of the microscope. Refer to your textbook to review the basic description, location, and function of each tissue type, and then locate some examples of each tissue type on the microscope slide. Carefully study each slide and answer the questions given at the end of each tissue section.

By the end of this laboratory exercise, you should be able to list the physical characteristics, location, and function of the tissue types encountered at the stations. You should also be able to draw any of the tissue types from today's laboratory exercise.

The following outline will help in organizing the information from today and should be useful in studying for examinations.

| Exercise 5.1 | Simple Squamous Epithelium |

Instructions: Observe the slide and refer to your textbook to answer the following questions:

1. Describe the physical characteristics of simple squamous cells.

   _____

   _____

   _____

   _____

2. Where in the human body can the simple squamous epithelium be found?

   _____

   _____

   _____

   _____

3. What functions does this type of epithelium perform?

   _____

   _____

   _____

   _____

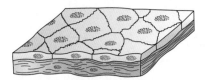

Figure 5.1

Stratified Squamous Epithelium

Instructions: Observe the slide and refer to your textbook to answer the following questions:

1. Describe the physical characteristics of both keratinized and nonkeratinized stratified squamous epithelia.

_____

_____

_____

_____

2. Where in the human body is the stratified squamous epithelium (keratinized and nonkeratinized) located?

_____

_____

_____

_____

3. What functions does this type of epithelium perform?

_____

_____

_____

_____

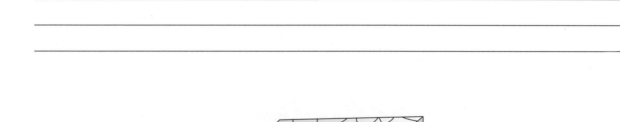

Figure 5.2

| Exercise 5.3 | Simple Cuboidal Epithelium |

Instructions: Observe the slide and refer to your textbook to answer the following questions:

1. Describe the physical characteristics of cuboidal cells.

_____

_____

_____

_____

2. Where in the human body is the simple cuboidal epithelium located?

_____

_____

_____

_____

3. What functions does this type of epithelium perform?

_____

_____

_____

_____

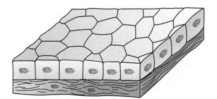

Figure 5.3

Simple Columnar Epithelium

Instructions: Observe the slide and refer to your textbook to answer the following questions:

1. Describe the physical characteristics of simple columnar epithelium.

   _____

   _____

   _____

   _____

2. Where in the human body is the simple columnar epithelium located?

   _____

   _____

   _____

   _____

3. What functions does this type of epithelium perform?

   _____

   _____

   _____

   _____

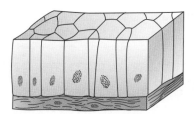

Figure 5.4

Pseudostratified Ciliated Columnar Epithelium

Exercise 5.5

Instructions: Observe the slide and refer to your textbook to answer the following questions:

1. Describe the physical characteristics of pseudostratified epithelium.

   _____

   _____

   _____

   _____

2. Why does this epithelial tissue appear to be "stratified"?

   _____

   _____

   _____

   _____

3. Where in the human body is the pseudostratified columnar epithelium (ciliated and nonciliated) located?

   _____

   _____

   _____

   _____

4. What functions does this type of epithelium perform?

   _____

   _____

   _____

   _____

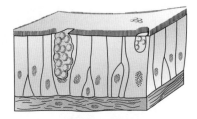

Figure 5.5

Transitional Epithelium

Instructions: Observe the slide and refer to your textbook to answer the following questions:

1. Describe the physical characteristics of transitional epithelium.

_____

_____

_____

_____

2. Where in the human body can the transitional epithelium be found?

_____

_____

_____

_____

3. What functions does this type of epithelium perform?

_____

_____

_____

_____

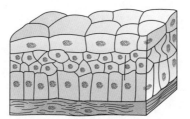

Figure 5.6

Dense Regular Connective Tissue

Exercise 5.7

Instructions: Observe the slide and refer to your textbook to answer the following questions:

1. Describe the physical characteristics of dense regular connective tissue.

   _____

   _____

   _____

   _____

2. Name the type of cells that synthesize the collagen fibers.

   _____

   _____

   _____

   _____

3. Where in the human body is the dense regular connective tissue located?

   _____

   _____

   _____

   _____

4. What functions does this type of tissue perform?

_____

_____

_____

_____

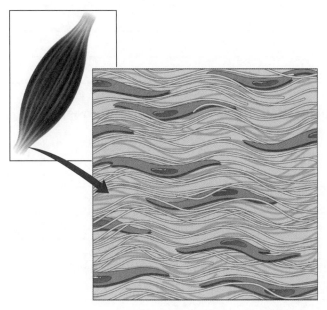

Figure 5.7

Exercise 5.8

Dense Irregular Connective Tissue

Instructions: Observe the slide and refer to your textbook to answer the following questions:

1. Describe the physical characteristics of dense irregular connective tissue.

_____

_____

_____

_____

2. What is the difference between the terms "regular" and "irregular" when applied to connective tissue?

_____

_____

_____

_____

3. Where in the human body is the dense irregular connective tissue located?

_____

_____

_____

_____

4. What functions does this type of connective tissue perform?

_____

_____

_____

_____

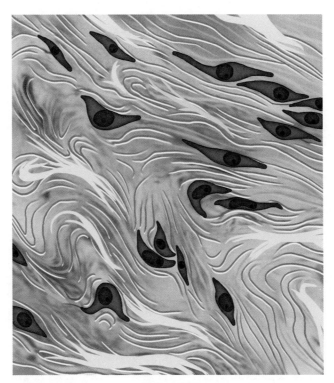

Figure 5.8

Hyaline Cartilage

Exercise 5.9

Instructions: Observe the slide and refer to your textbook to answer the following questions:

1. Describe the physical characteristics of hyaline cartilage and indicate what type of cells produce the matrix.

_____

_____

_____

_____

2. What is a lacuna?

_____

_____

_____

_____

3. Where in the adult human body is the hyaline cartilage located? Where in the human embryo is it found?

_____

_____

_____

_____

4. What functions does hyaline cartilage perform?

_____

_____

_____

_____

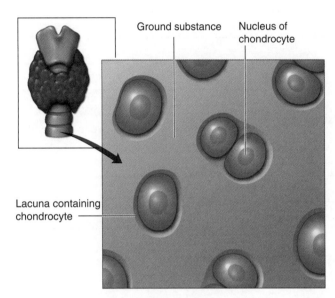

Ground substance   Nucleus of
                    chondrocyte

Lacuna containing
chondrocyte

Figure 5.9

Exercise 5.10	Elastic Cartilage

Instructions: Observe the slide and refer to your textbook to answer the following questions:

1. Describe the physical characteristics of elastic cartilage.

_____

_____

_____

_____

2. What type of cells synthesize elastic fibers?

_____

_____

_____

_____

3. Where in the human body is the elastic cartilage located?

_____

_____

_____

_____

4. What functions does elastic cartilage perform?

_____

_____

_____

_____

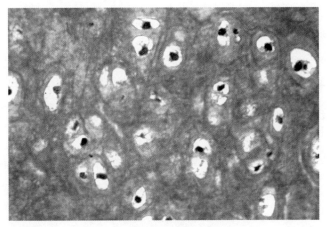

Figure 5.10

Exercise 5.11

Bone (Osseous Tissue)

Instructions: Observe the slide of bone tissue and use your textbook to answer the following questions:

1. What cell makes the bony matrix?

_____

_____

_____

_____

2. Describe the structure of the bone tissue at the diaphysis (shaft) and compare this to the epiphyseal end of a typical long bone.

_____

_____

_____

_____

3. What is the functional significance of the lacuna?

_____

_____

_____

_____

Skeletal Muscle

Instructions: Observe the slide and refer to your textbook to answer the following questions:

1. Describe the physical characteristics of skeletal muscle tissue.

_____

_____

_____

_____

2. Which division of the nervous system (voluntary or involuntary) controls skeletal muscle tissue?

_____

_____

_____

_____

3. Name the proteins that give the striated appearance in skeletal muscle cells and label the striations in Figure 5.11.

_____

_____

_____

_____

4. What functions does skeletal muscle tissue perform?

_____

_____

_____

_____

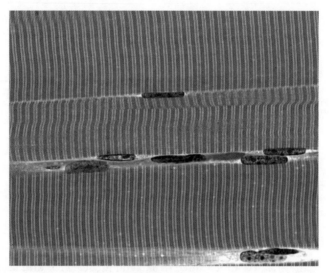

Figure 5.11

Cardiac Muscle

Instructions: Observe the slide and refer to your textbook to answer the following questions:

1. Describe the physical characteristics of cardiac muscle tissue.

   _____

   _____

   _____

   _____

2. Which division of the nervous system (voluntary or involuntary) controls cardiac muscle tissue?

   _____

   _____

   _____

   _____

3. Name the proteins that give the striated appearance in cardiac muscle cells.

   _____

   _____

   _____

   _____

4. What functions does cardiac muscle tissue perform?

_____

_____

_____

_____

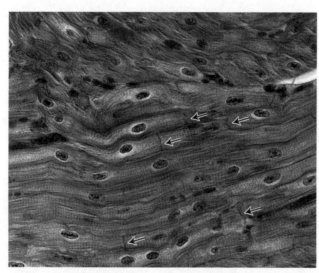

Figure 5.12 Cardiac muscle.

Smooth Muscle

Instructions: Observe the slide and refer to your textbook to answer the following questions:

1. Describe the physical characteristics of smooth muscle tissue.

   _____

   _____

   _____

   _____

2. Name the two major proteins present in smooth muscle cells that allow them to contract.

   _____

   _____

   _____

   _____

3. When smooth muscle cells contract, what happens (dilation or constriction) to blood vessel diameter?

   _____

   _____

   _____

   _____

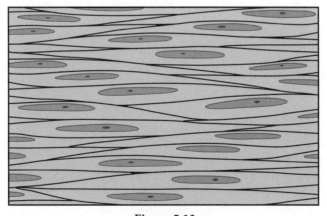

Figure 5.13

Exercise 5.15   Neural Tissue

Instructions: Observe the slide and refer to your textbook to answer the following questions:

1. What are the divisions of the nervous system?

   _____

   _____

   _____

   _____

2. Which two organs comprise the central division of the nervous system?

   _____

   _____

   _____

   _____

3. What function(s) does nervous tissue perform?

   _____

   _____

   _____

   _____

4. Label the following structures in Figure 5.14.
- ▪ Axon
- ▪ Cell body
- ▪ Dendrites
- ▪ Synaptic terminal

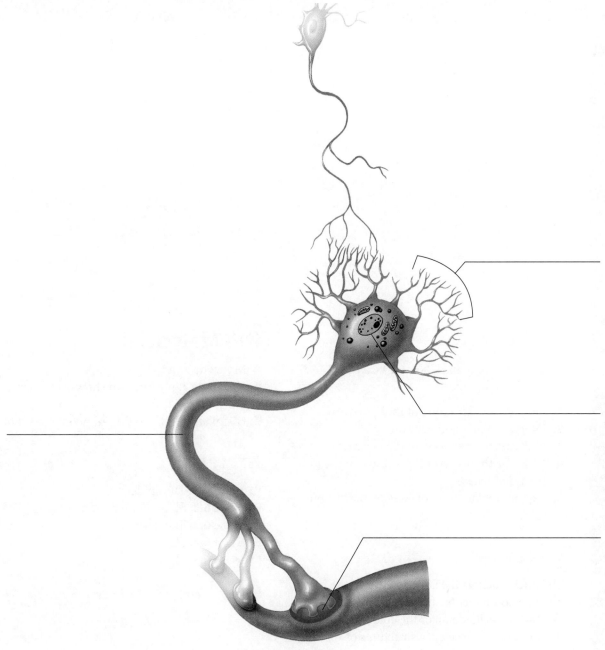

Figure 5.14

The Integumentary System

Objectives

After completing this laboratory exercise, students will be able to:

1. Describe the structure of the epidermis.
2. Describe skin pigmentation.
3. Describe the structure of the dermis.
4. Describe the accessory structures of the skin (hair and nails).
5. Explain the function of sweat glands in the skin.

Overview

The integument is the largest organ of the body. The two components of the integument are the skin, which is made up of the epidermis and the dermis, and the accessory structures of the skin such as sensory organs, glands, hair, and nails. In this lab, you will encounter the skin at the gross and microscopic level.

Lab Materials

- Model of skin
- Histological preparation showing the layers of the epidermis
- Histological preparation of pigmented skin

Exercises

Exercise 6.1: The epidermis
Exercise 6.2: Skin pigmentation
Exercise 6.3: The dermis
Exercise 6.4: Hair
Exercise 6.5: Nails

Estimated lab time: 60 minutes

The Epidermis

Instructions: The epidermis is composed of several layers. In Figure 6.1, label the following layers of the epidermis. Then observe the microscopic preparation of the epidermis and find each of the layers.

- Stratum corneum
- Stratum lucidum
- Stratum granulosum
- Stratum spinosum
- Stratum basale

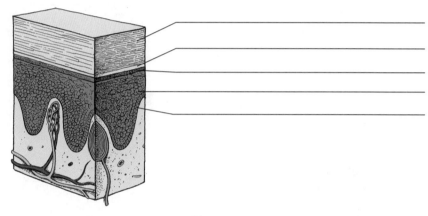

Figure 6.1

Study Questions

1. Where would you find stem cells and dead keratinized cells?

   _____

   _____

   _____

2. What is the function of keratin?

   _____

   _____

   _____

| Exercise 6.2 | Skin Pigmentation |

1. Describe how melanin is dispersed from the melanocyte to the epidermal cells in Figure 6.2.

_____

_____

_____

2. What is the relationship between the amount of melanin produced and protection from ultraviolet radiation?

_____

_____

_____

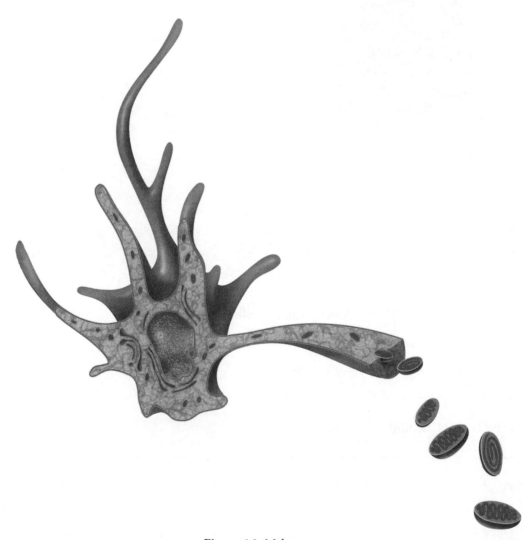

Figure 6.2 Melanocyte

Study Questions

1. What is the function of melanin?

_____

_____

_____

2. Describe what causes the difference in skin pigmentation from one person to the other.

_____

_____

_____

Instructions: Observe a microscopic preparation of pigmented skin and draw what you see.

Exercise 6.3

The Dermis

Instructions: Identify the papillary dermis and the reticular dermis in Figure 6.3. List the accessory glands and structures found in the reticular dermis.

▪ Accessory glands and structures in the reticular dermis:

_____

_____

_____

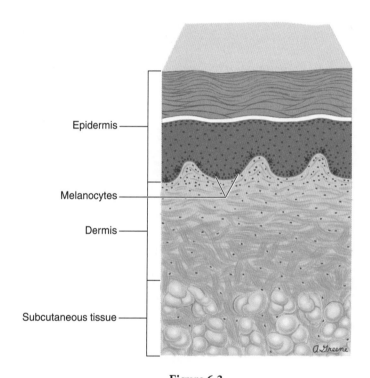

Epidermis ——

Melanocytes ——

Dermis ——

Subcutaneous tissue ——

Figure 6.3

Hair

Instructions: Label the following structures in Figure 6.4:

- Hair bulb
- Sebaceous gland
- Arrector pili
- Hair follicle

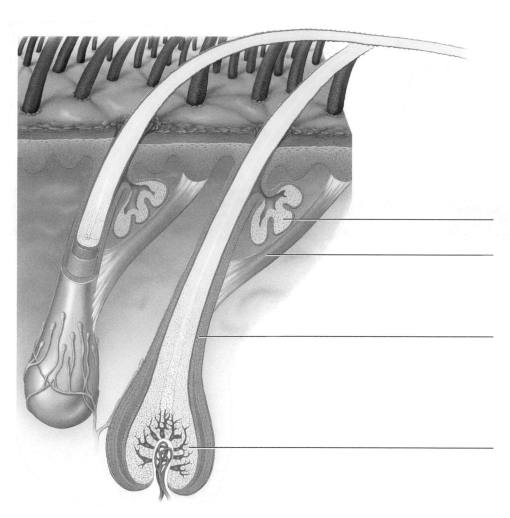

Figure 6.4

Study Questions

1. What is responsible for hair color?

_____

_____

_____

2. Why does some hair turn white?

_____

_____

_____

Nails

Exercise 6.5

Instructions: Label the following structures in Figure 6.5:

- Nail plate
- Nail bed
- Nail fold
- Hyponychium
- Lunula
- Eponychium
- Nail matrix
- Nail root

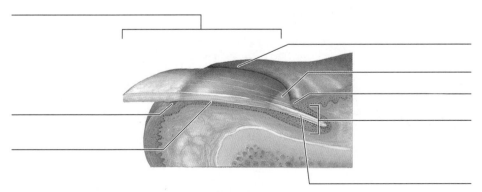

Figure 6.5

The Skeletal System

Objectives

After completing this laboratory exercise, students will be able to identify:

1. Axial skeleton
   - Bones of the skull
   - Selected foramina of the skull
   - Sutures and sinuses in the skull
   - Bones of the vertebrae
   - Sternum, ribs, and hyoid bones
2. Appendicular skeleton—the bones and the boney features of the
   - Pectoral girdle
   - Pelvic girdle
   - Upper limb
   - Lower limb
3. Articulations
   - Identify examples of synarthrotic, amphiarthrotic, and diarthrotic joints.
   - Name the bones and boney features that articulate at each of the identified joints.
   - Describe the motions allowed at identified joints.
   - Describe the pathology of selected joint disorders.

Overview

The purpose of this laboratory exercise is to familiarize the student with an understanding of the major structures of the skeletal system. Students are expected to identify the major bones and several major bony landmarks.

The laboratory exercise is subdivided into three sections. The axial skeleton section appears first, which consists of the bones of the skull, the vertebrae, and the thoracic cage. This is followed by the appendicular skeleton section, which consists of the bones of the upper and lower limbs. The final section of this exercise is the joints or articulations.

Lab Materials

- Prepared slide of cross-section of osseous tissue

Each group should have the following models:

- Articulated skeleton
- Fully disarticulated skeleton
- Knee, elbow, shoulder, hip, wrist, and ankle joints

Exercises

The axial skeleton
- **7.1:** Skull: Cranial bones
- **7.2:** Skull: The sphenoid bone
- **7.3:** Skull: The ethmoid bone
- **7.4:** Skull: Facial bones
- **7.5:** Skull: Mandible
- **7.6:** Skull: Inferior view
- **7.7:** Skull: Sutures
- **7.8:** The vertebral column
- **7.9:** The cervical vertebrae
- **7.10:** The thoracic vertebrae
- **7.11:** The lumbar vertebrae
- **7.12:** The sacrum and coccyx
- **7.13:** The sternum and ribs
- **7.14:** Osseous tissue

The appendicular skeleton
- **7.15:** The scapula and clavicle
- **7.16:** The humerus
- **7.17:** The radius and ulna
- **7.18:** The bones of the hand
- **7.19:** The bones of the hip
- **7.20:** The femur
- **7.21:** The tibia and fibula
- **7.22:** The bones of the foot

Joints/articulations
- **7.23:** Movements allowed by joints
- **7.24:** The joints of the skull
- **7.25:** The shoulder joint
- **7.26:** Elbow joint
- **7.27:** Joints of the forearm
- **7.28:** Joints of the hand
- **7.29:** The hip joint
- **7.30:** The knee joint
- **7.31:** The ankle
- **7.32:** Joints of the vertebral column

Estimated lab time: 2 hours

THE AXIAL SKELETON

In this section, refer to your textbook and the models to identify the structures indicated.

Skull: Cranial Bones

Instructions: Identify and label the following structures in Figure 7.1:

▪ Frontal
▪ Parietal
▪ Occipital
▪ Temporal
  ☐ Mastoid process
  ☐ Styloid process
  ☐ Zygomatic process
  ☐ External acoustic meatus

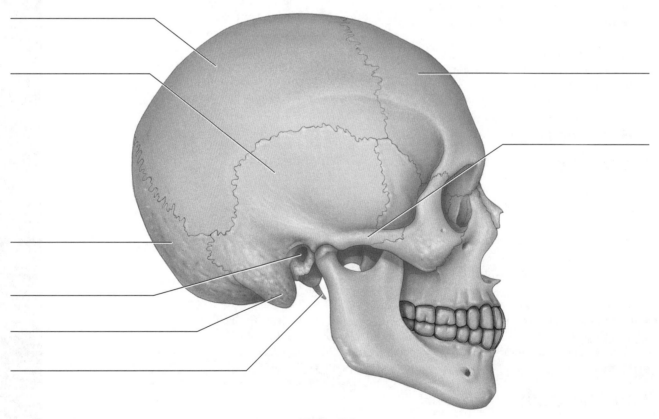

Figure 7.1

Skull: The Sphenoid Bone

Instructions: Identify and label the following structures in Figures 7.2 and 7.3:

- Greater wing
- Lesser wing
- Sella turcica
- Optic canal

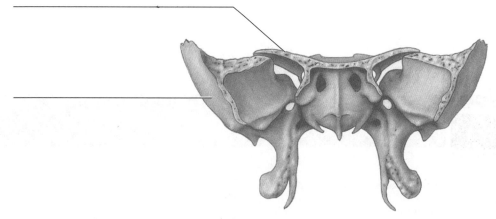

Figure 7.2

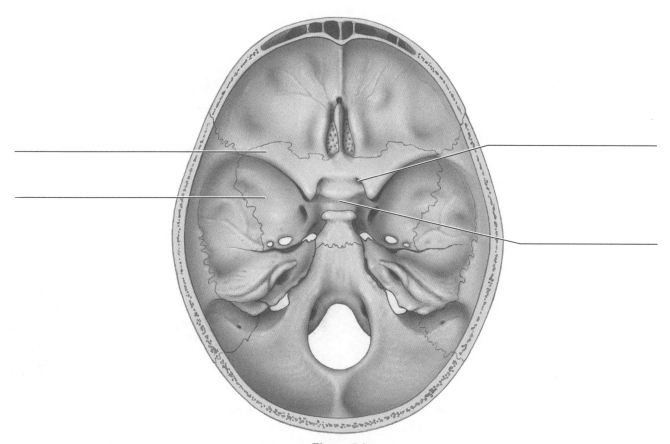

Figure 7.3

Study Questions

1. Why is the sphenoid bone commonly referred to as the "keystone" of the skull?

_____

_____

| Exercise 7.3 | Skull: The Ethmoid Bone |

Instructions: Identify and label the following structures in Figure 7.4:

◼ Cribriform plate (use twice)
◼ Cristi galli (use twice)
◼ Ethmoid sinuses

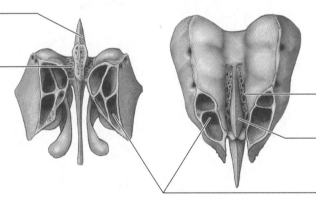

Figure 7.4

Skull: Facial Bones

Instructions: Identify and label the following structures in Figure 7.5:

- Zygomatic bone
- Nasal bone
- Lacrimal bone
- Maxilla
- Infraorbital foramen
- Alveolar process
- Mandible
  - ☐ Mental foramen
  - ☐ Alveolar process

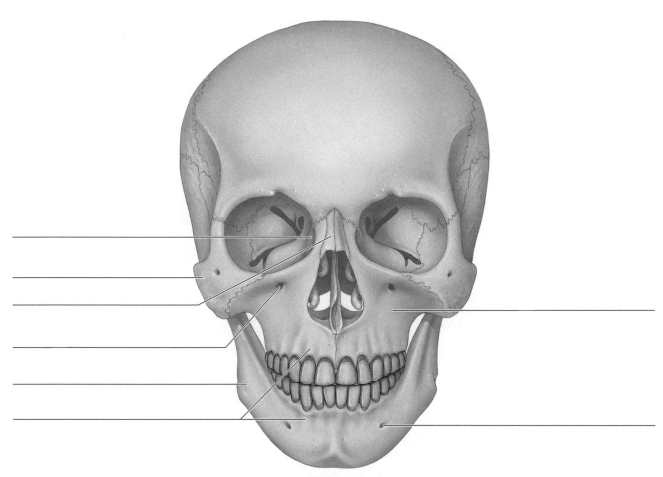

Figure 7.5

| Exercise 7.5 | Skull: Mandible |

Instructions: Identify and label the following in Figure 7.6:

- Body
- Ramus
- Angle
- Mental foramen
- Alveolar process
- Coronoid process
- Condylar process

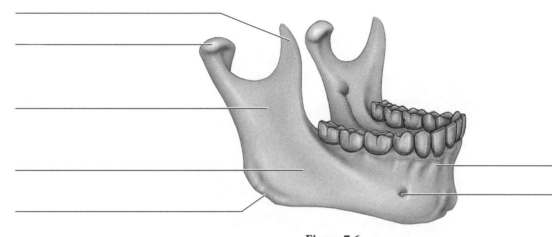

Figure 7.6

Skull: Inferior View

Instructions: Identify and label the following structures in Figure 7.7:

- Temporal bone
- Occipital bone
- Occipital condyles
- External occipital protuberance
- External acoustic meatus
- Stylomastoid foramen
- Carotid canal
- Jugular foramen
- Foramen magnum
- Vomer

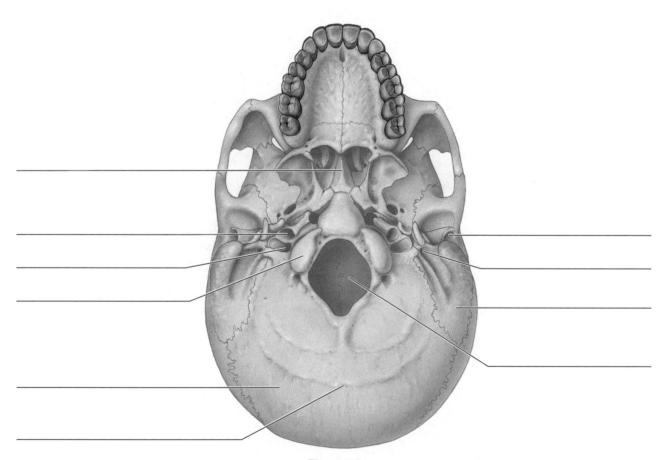

Figure 7.7

Exercise 7.7   Skull: Sutures

Instructions: Identify and label the following structures in Figure 7.8:

- Coronal suture
- Lambdoid suture
- Squamous suture
- Occipitomastoid suture

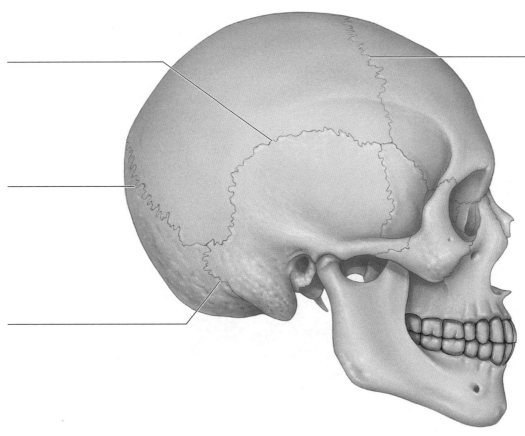

Figure 7.8

The Vertebral Column

Instructions: Identify and label the following regions of the vertebral column in Figure 7.9:

- Cervical region
- Thoracic region
- Lumbar region
- Sacrum
- Coccyx

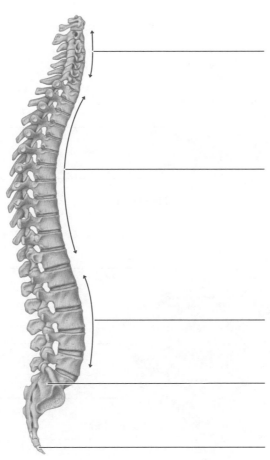

Figure 7.9

The Cervical Vertebrae

Exercise 7.9

Instructions: Identify and label the following items in Figures 7.10 and 7.11:

- Transverse foramen
- Superior articular facet
- Bifid spinous process
- C1 (atlas)
- C2 (axis)
- Dens

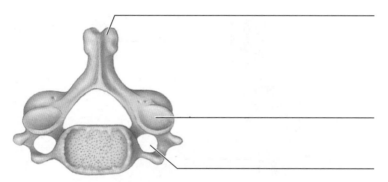

Figure 7.10

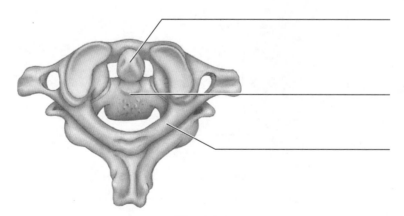

Figure 7.11

The Thoracic Vertebrae

Instructions: Identify and label the following items in Figures 7.12 and 7.13:

- Superior articular process
- Costal facets
    - ☐ Pedicle
    - ☐ Lamina
    - ☐ Transverse process
    - ☐ Spinous process
    - ☐ Vertebral arch

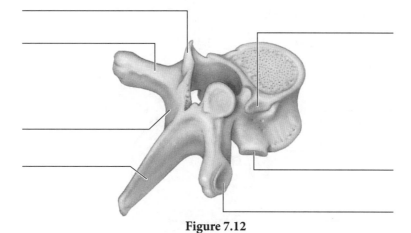

Figure 7.12

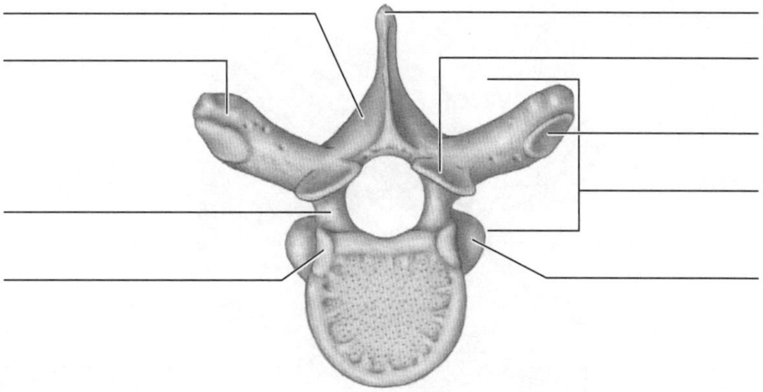

Figure 7.13

Exercise 7.11

The Lumbar Vertebrae

Instructions: Identify and label the following items in Figures 7.14 and 7.15:

■ Superior articular facet
- ☐ Pedicle
- ☐ Lamina
- ☐ Transverse process
- ☐ Spinous process
- ☐ Vertebral arch

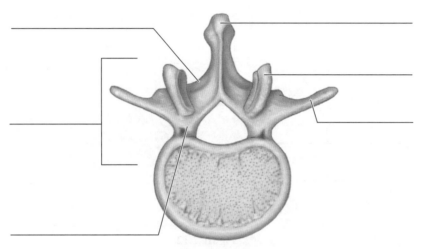

Figure 7.14

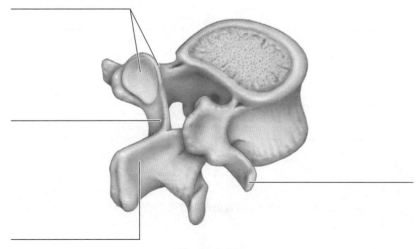

Figure 7.15

The Sacrum and Coccyx

Instructions: Identify and label the following items in Figure 7.16:

- Sacrum
- Sacral foramen
- Sacral canal
- Lateral sacral crest
- Median sacral crest
- Intermediate sacral crest
- Coccyx

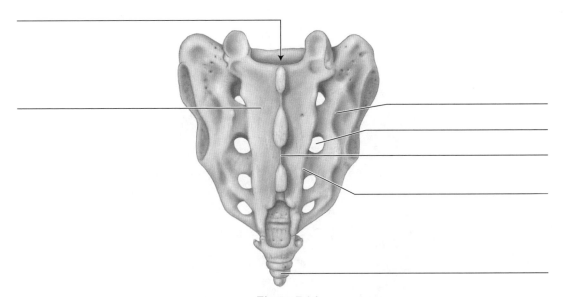

Figure 7.16

Exercise 7.13   The Sternum and Ribs

Instructions: Identify and label the following items in Figure 7.17:

- Manubrium
- Sternum (body)
- Xiphoid process
  - ☐ True ribs (1 to 7)
  - ☐ False ribs (8 to 10)
  - ☐ Floating ribs (11 and 12)
  - ☐ Costal cartilage

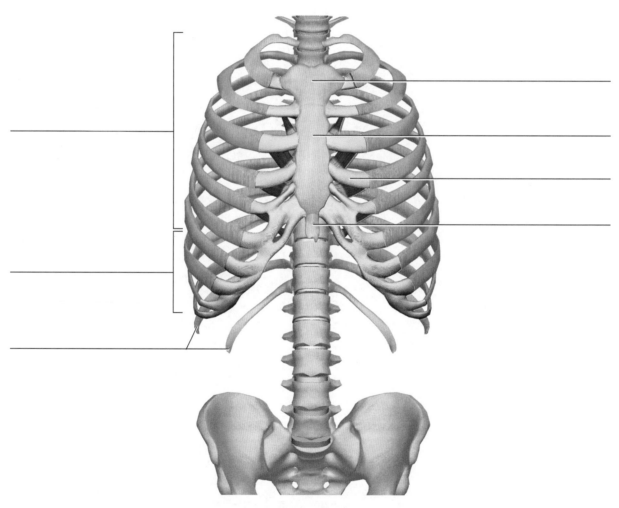

Figure 7.17

Osseous Tissue

Instructions: Observe a prepared slide of osseous tissue cross section. Refer to your textbook and the prepared slide to identify the following structures in Figure 7.18:

- Canaliculi
- Central canal
- Lamellae
- Lacunae
- Osteocyte
- Spongy bone
- Compact bone

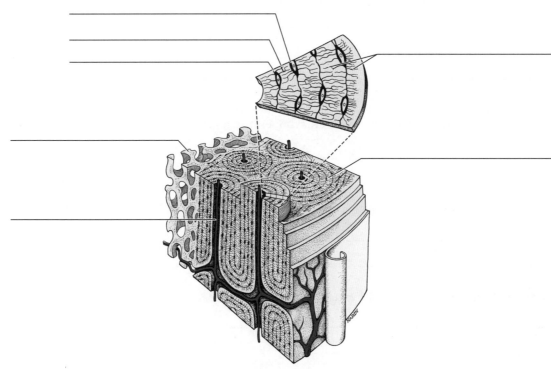

Figure 7.18

Study Questions

1. List the eight bones of the cranium AND classify them as long, short, flat, or irregular.

Cranial Bone(s)	Classification
1.	
2.	
3.	
4.	
5.	
6.	
7.	
8.	

2. What type of joint is formed when any two cranial bones fuse together?

_____

_____

3. Which vital organ does the cranium protect?

_____

_____

4. Which structure funnels sound into the external auditory meatus?

_____

_____

5. Which bones form the nasal septum?

_____

_____

6. What is "cheek" bone?

_____

_____

7. Name the two bones that form the sagittal suture.

   _____

   _____

8. What are "soft spots" in a baby's head?

   _____

   _____

9. What purpose/function do sinuses serve in the skull?

   _____

   _____

10. Which cavity does fluid from sinuses drain into?

    _____

    _____

11. What types of structures pass through the various foramina of the skull?

    _____

    _____

12. Which structure extends through the foramen magnum in a living human?

    _____

    _____

13. Name the two processes of the temporal bone that the stylomastoid foramen is located between.

    _____

    _____

14. What happens to pipe cleaners as they are simultaneously passed through the right and left optic canals?

    _____

    _____

15. List the different vertebrae in the spinal column and describe the distinguishing characteristics for each type of vertebra.

    _____

    _____

    _____

16. Name the two bones that the C1 (atlas) articulates with?

_____

_____

17. The vertebral body of C1 is absent. Where do you think the body of the atlas is?

_____

_____

18. What is the name of the structure located between the bodies of adjacent vertebrae?

_____

_____

THE APPENDICULAR SKELETON

In this section, refer to your textbook and the models to identify the structures indicated.

| Exercise 7.15 | The Scapula and Clavicle |

Instructions: Identify and label the following items in Figure 7.19:

■ Sternal end of clavicle
■ Acromial end of clavicle

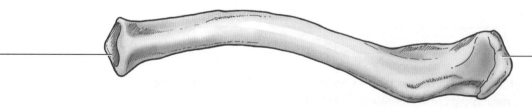

Figure 7.19

Instructions: Identify and label the following items in Figures 7.20 and 7.21:

- Spine
- Acromion process
- Coracoid process
- Supraspinous fossa
- Infraspinous fossa
- Glenoid cavity
- Subscapular fossa
- Medial border

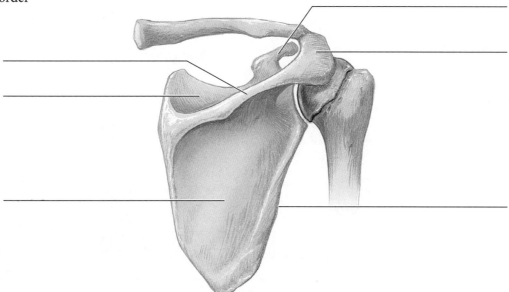

Figure 7.20

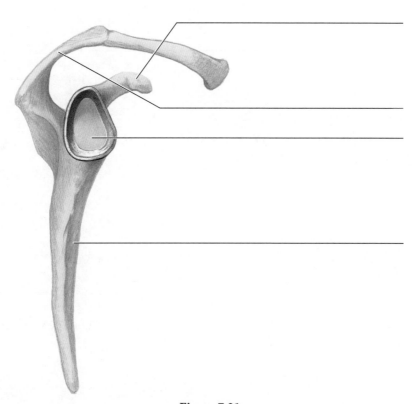

Figure 7.21

Exercise 7.16	The Humerus

Instructions: Identify and label the following items in Figures 7.22 and 7.23:

- Head
- Anatomical neck
- Surgical neck
- Greater tubercle
- Lesser tubercle
- Intertubercular groove
- Medial epicondyle
- Lateral epicondyle
- Deltoid tuberosity
- Capitulum
- Trochlea
- Coronoid fossa
- Olecranon fossa

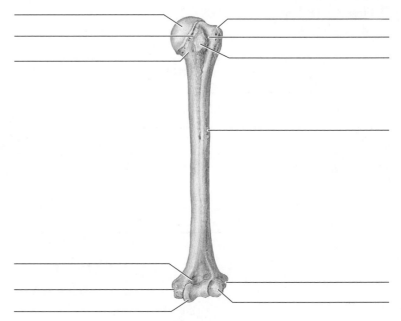

Figure 7.22

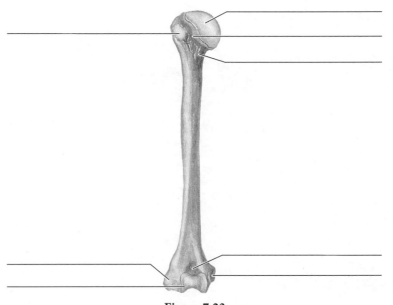

Figure 7.23

The Radius and Ulna

Instructions: Identify and label the following items in Figures 7.24 and 7.25:

- **Radius**
  - ☐ Head (proximal end)
  - ☐ Styloid process (distal end)
  - ☐ Radial tuberosity
- **Ulna**
  - ☐ Olecranon process
  - ☐ Trochlear notch
  - ☐ Coronoid process
  - ☐ Styloid process of ulna
  - ☐ Head (distal end)

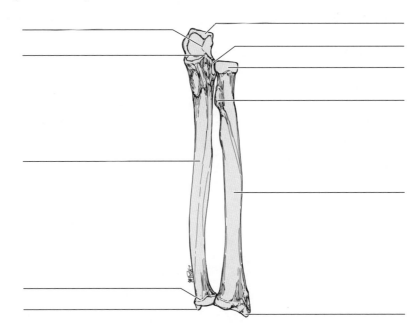

Figure 7.24

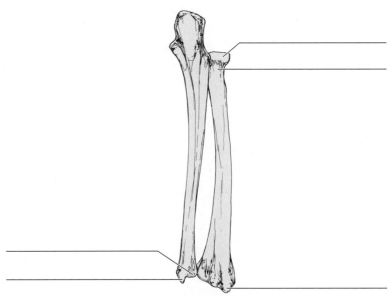

Figure 7.25

Exercise 7.18 | The Bones of the Hand

Instructions: Identify and label the following items in Figure 7.26:

■ **Carpal Bones**
- ☐ Trapezoid
- ☐ Trapezium
- ☐ Scaphoid
- ☐ Capitate
- ☐ Hamate
- ☐ Pisiform
- ☐ Triquetral
- ☐ Lunate

■ **Metacarpals**
- ☐ I
- ☐ II
- ☐ III
- ☐ IV
- ☐ V

■ **Phalanges**
- ☐ Proximal
- ☐ Middle
- ☐ Distal

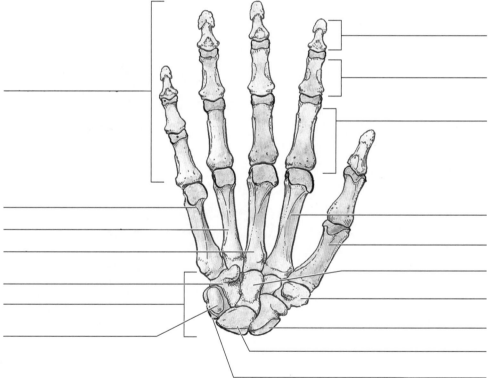

Figure 7.26

The Bones of the Hip

Exercise 7.19

Instructions: Identify and label the following items in Figures 7.27 and 7.28:

- **Ilium**
  - ☐ Iliac crest
  - ☐ Anterior superior iliac spine
  - ☐ Acetabulum
- **Ischium**
  - ☐ Ischial tuberosity
- **Pubis**
  - ☐ Pubic symphysis
  - ☐ Pubic arch
  - ☐ Obturator foramen

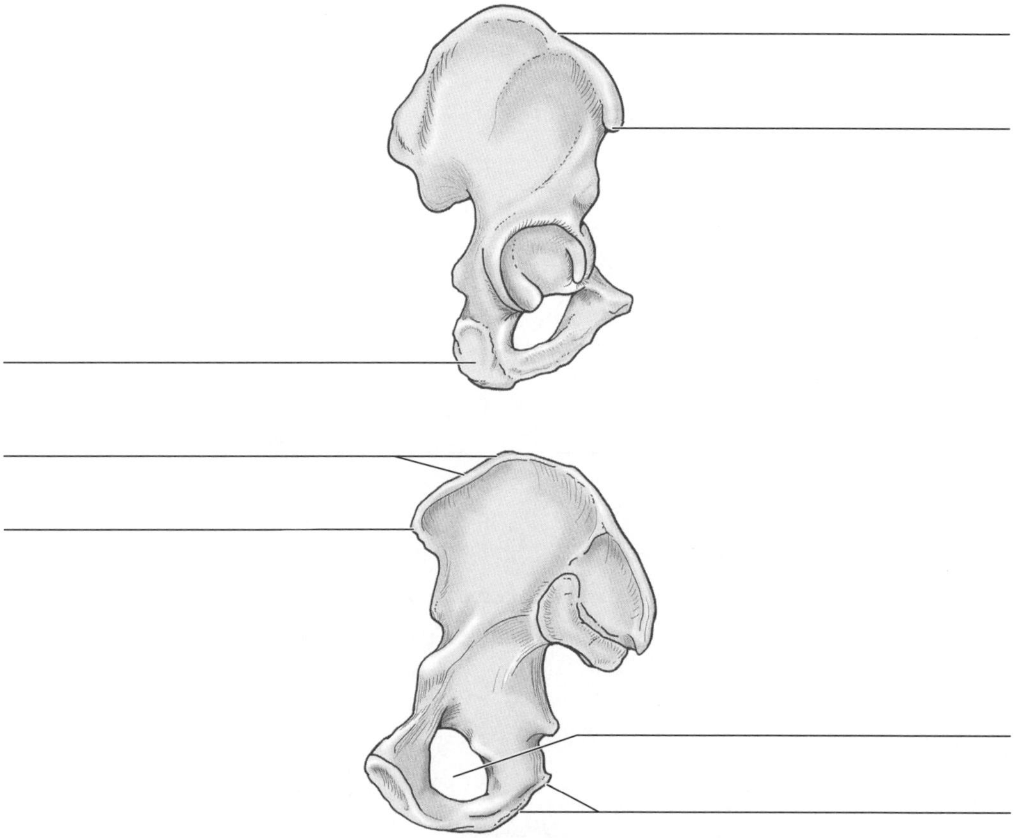

Figure 7.27

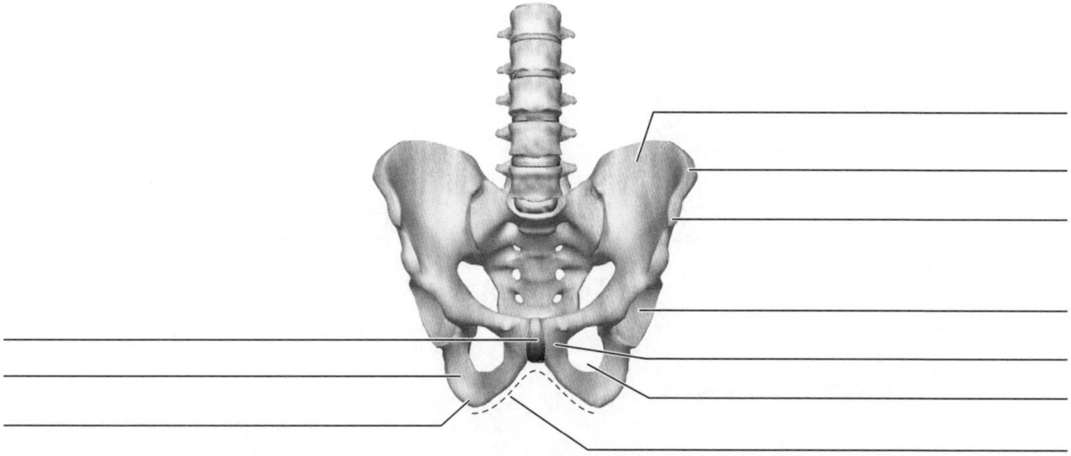

Figure 7.28

Exercise 7.20

The Femur

Instructions: Identify and label the following items in Figure 7.29:

- Head
- Neck
- Greater trochanter
- Lesser trochanter
- Gluteal tuberosity
- Linea aspera
- Medial condyle
- Lateral condyle
- Intercondylar fossa
- Lateral epicondyle
- Medial epicondyle

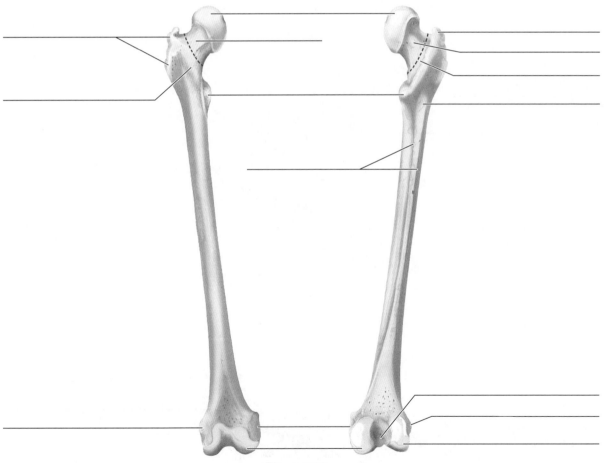

Figure 7.29

The Tibia and Fibula

Instructions: Identify and label the following items in Figures 7.30 and 7.31:

- ▪ **Tibia**
  - ☐ Medial condyle
  - ☐ Lateral condyle
  - ☐ Tibial tuberosity
  - ☐ Medial malleolus
- ▪ **Fibula**
  - ☐ Head
  - ☐ Lateral malleolus

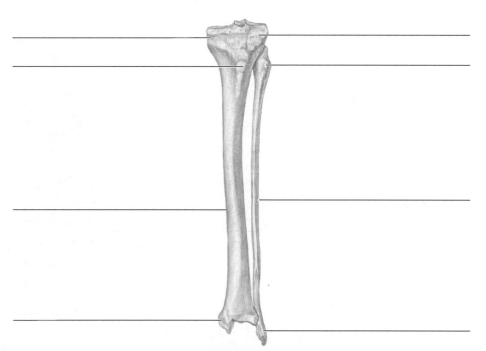

Figure 7.30

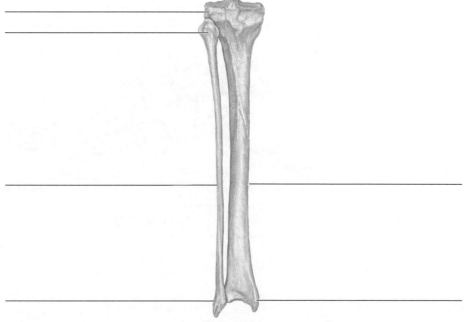

Figure 7.31

The Bones of the Foot

Exercise 7.22

Instructions: Identify and label the following items in Figures 7.32 and 7.33:

- **Tarsal bones**
  - ☐ Talus
    - ☐ Trochlea of talus
  - ☐ Calcaneus
    - ☐ Calcaneal tuberosity
  - ☐ Cuboid
  - ☐ Lateral cuneiform
  - ☐ Medial cuneiform
  - ☐ Intermediate cuneiform
  - ☐ Navicular
- **Metatarsal bones**
- **Phalanges**
  - ☐ Proximal
  - ☐ Middle
  - ☐ Distal

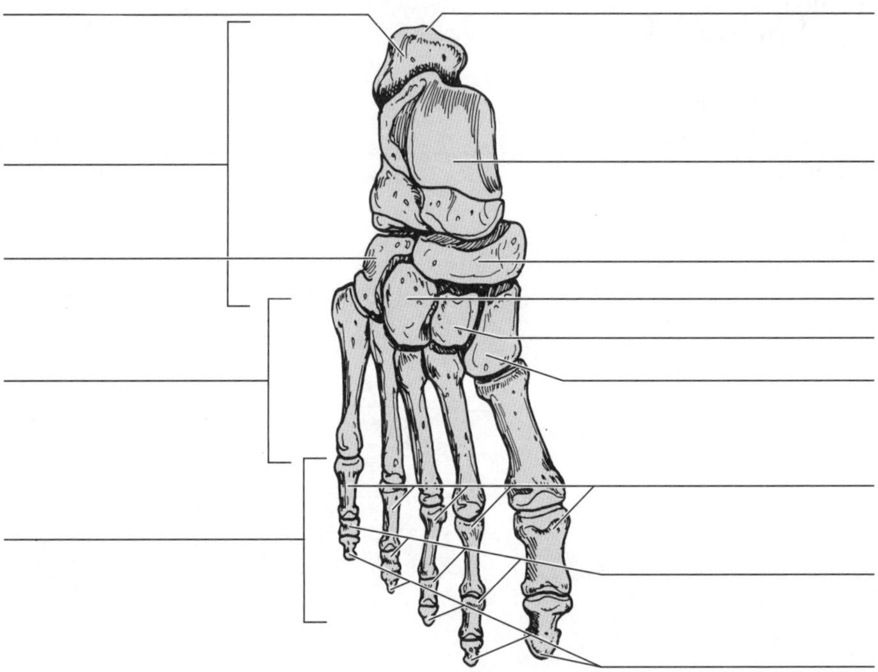

Figure 7.32

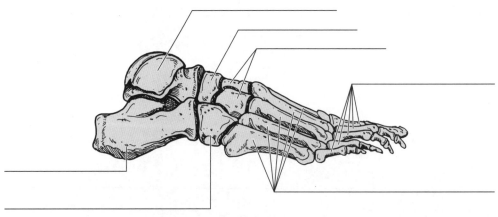

Figure 7.33

Study Questions

1. Describe the function of the pectoral girdle and name the two bones comprising it.

    _____

    _____

2. Name the bones that the clavicle articulates with at the medial and lateral ends.

    _____

    _____

3. Which bones are commonly called the "collar bone" and the "shoulder blade"?

    _____

    _____

4. Which surface feature of the scapula does the head of the humerus articulate with?

    _____

    _____

5. Explain what clinical significance the term "surgical" neck of the humerus connotes.

    _____

    _____

6. Name the prominent arm muscle, the tendon of which is located in the intertubercular groove.

    _____

    _____

7. Determine whether the ulna is medial or lateral to the radius.

    _____

    _____

8. What happens to the palm of the hand during supination and pronation?

    _____

    _____

9. Which bone (radius or ulna) is moving during the process of pronation and supination?

    _____

    _____

10. Which types of bones (long/short/flat/irregular) are the carpal bones, metacarpal bones, and phalanges?

_____

_____

11. Write the common names for each digit I to V.

_____

_____

12. What boney processes form your most proximal row of knuckles?

_____

_____

13. Which of these bones is most commonly broken when you fall?

_____

_____

14. Explain the derivative of the word "acetabulum" from Latin or Greek by referring to a medical dictionary and then describe the shape of the acetabulum in the skeleton.

_____

_____

15. When seated, what boney process of the ischium is all your upper body weight directed upon?

_____

_____

16. Describe the anatomical differences between the male and female pubic arch.

_____

_____

17. Explain the derivative of the word "trochanter" by referring to a medical dictionary.

_____

_____

18. Name all the boney surfaces that make up the "hip joint."

_____

_____

19. Which bone in the lower part of the leg (tibia or fibula) does the medial and lateral condyle of the femur articulate with?

_____

_____

20. Is the position of the fibula medial or lateral to the tibia?

_____

_____

21. Explain the derivative of the word "malleolus" by referring to a medical dictionary.

_____

_____

22. When "kneeling," all the weight of the upper part of the body is directed upon which process of the tibia?

_____

_____

JOINTS/ARTICULATIONS

In this section, refer to your textbook and the models to identify the different types of joint structures and to describe the movements allowed by each joint.

| Exercise 7.23 | Movements Allowed by Joints |

Instructions: Define and describe the types of movements listed. Provide an example of where each movement can be demonstrated.

▪ Flexion

_____

_____

_____

▪ Extension

_____

_____

_____

▪ Hyperextension

_____

_____

_____

▪ Adduction

_____

_____

_____

▪ Abduction

_____

_____

_____

▪ Circumduction

_____

_____

_____

▪ Rotation

_____

_____

_____

▪ Supination

_____

_____

■ Pronation

_____

_____

_____

■ Eversion

_____

_____

_____

■ Inversion

_____

_____

_____

The Joints of the Skull

Exercise 7.24

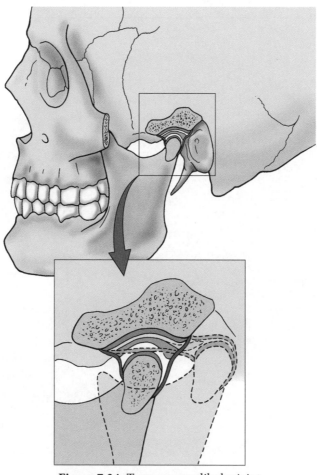

Figure 7.34 Temporomandibular joint

Study Questions

1. Name the only diarthrotic joint in the skull. Which bones articulate to form this joint?

_____

_____

2. Which type of synovial joint is the only diarthrotic joint in the skull?

_____

_____

3. What is the name of the bacterium that causes the condition called "lockjaw"?

_____

_____

4. What should you have done in the past 10 years to help prevent the occurrence of "lockjaw"?

_____

_____

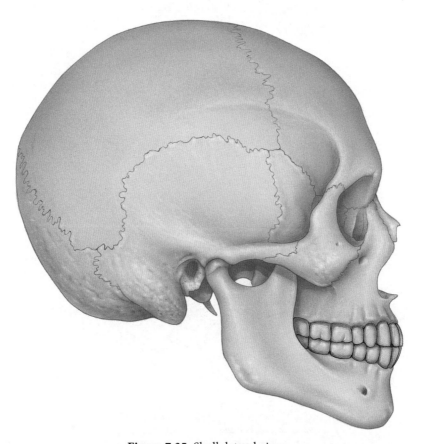

Figure 7.35 Skull, lateral view

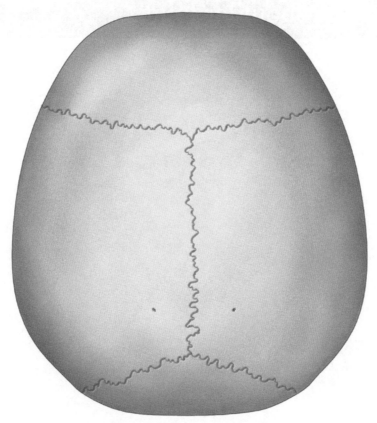

Figure 7.36 Skull, superior view

5. What type of joint is a sutural joint in the adult skull (synarthrotic, amphiarthrotic, diarthrotic)?

_____

_____

6. How much movement is allowed between bones at a sutural joint?

_____

_____

The Shoulder Joint

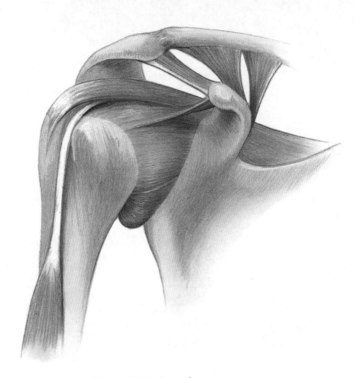

Figure 7.37 Scapula, anterior view

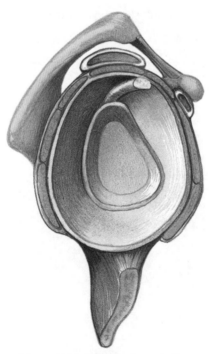

Figure 7.38 Scapula, lateral view

Study Questions

1. Name the bones and their processes that articulate at the shoulder joint.

   _____

   _____

2. What type of synovial joint is the shoulder (saddle, hinge, pivot, ball and socket, condyloid, gliding)?

   _____

   _____

3. List all types of movements allowed at the shoulder joint.

   _____

   _____

4. Name the four muscles involved in forming the "rotator cuff."

   _____

   _____

5. Which one of the rotator cuff muscles (tendons) is most often injured in baseball pitchers? Why?

   _____

   _____

Elbow Joint

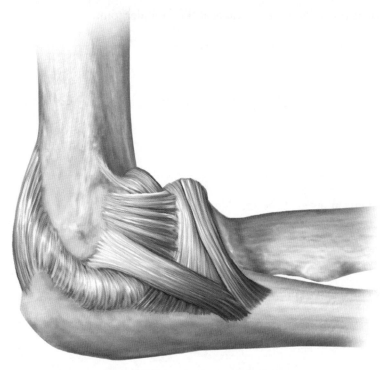

Figure 7.39 Left elbow, medial view

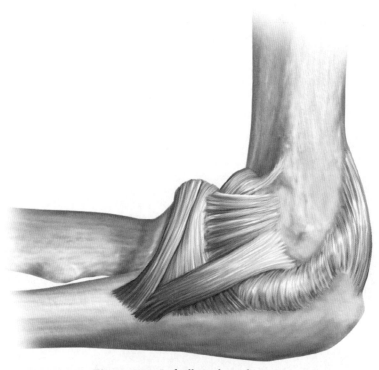

Figure 7.40 Left elbow, lateral view

Study Questions

1. Name the bones and their processes that articulate at the elbow joint.

   _____

   _____

2. What type of synovial joint is the elbow (saddle, hinge, pivot, ball and socket, condyloid, gliding)?

   _____

   _____

3. Name the type of motion that is permitted at the elbow joint.

   _____

   _____

4. What is the other name for "lateral epicondylitis"?

   _____

   _____

5. What type of synovial joint is formed between the head of the radius and the ulna (saddle, hinge, pivot, ball and socket, condyloid, gliding)?

   _____

   _____

| Exercise 7.27 | Joints of the Forearm |

Study Questions

1. Locate the following joints in Figure 7.41:

   a. Proximal radioulnar joint

   b. Distal radioulnar joint

2. What movements are possible by these joints?

   _____

   _____

3. What is the function of the interosseous membrane?

   _____

   _____

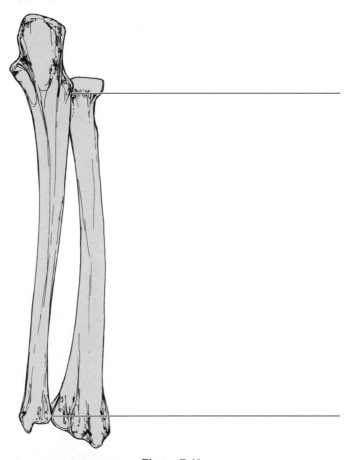

Figure 7.41

Joints of the Hand

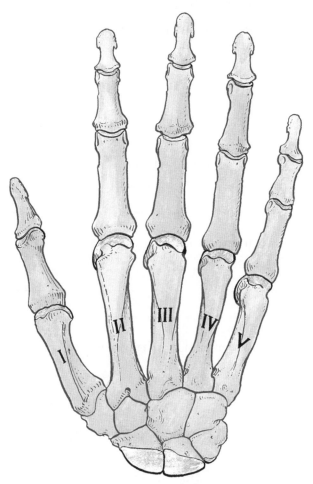

Figure 7.42 Right hand, dorsal view

Study Questions

1. Name the type of synovial joint and the motion(s) allowed between the following bones:

    a. Between the proximal phalanges and the middle phalanges

    _____

    _____

    b. Between the metacarpals and the proximal phalanges

    _____

    _____

    c. Between the distal ends of the radius and the carpal bones

    _____

    _____

2. When clenching your fist, what structures are formed by the distal heads of each metacarpal?

    _____

    _____

3. Define "arthritis" and explain why it is so painful, especially in joints like the hand.

    _____

    _____

4. Why does aspirin (or drugs like aspirin) relieve pain associated with arthritis?

    _____

    _____

The Hip Joint

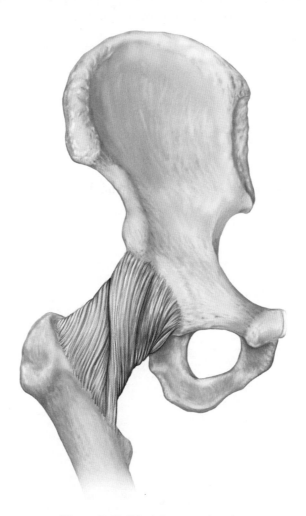

Figure 7.43 Hip joint, anterior view

Study Questions

1. Name the bones and processes of each bone forming the hip joint.

   _____

   _____

2. Describe what "subluxation" of the hip joint refers to.

   _____

   _____

3. An elderly lady falls and "breaks her hip." Name the most commonly broken bone and state the cause of it.

   _____

   _____

4. What is replaced during a "hip replacement?"

   _____

   _____

The Knee Joint

Study Questions

1. Name the bones and their associated structures that articulate at the knee joint.

   _____

   _____

2. Look at the model and Figure 7.44 and determine where the two menisci are located and indicate which of the two is firmly attached to a collateral ligament. Label these in Figure 7.44.

3. Name the microsurgical procedure to remove torn cartilage in the knee joint.

   _____

   _____

Instructions: In Figures 7.44 and 7.45, name and label all four of the ligaments that help stabilize the knee joint.

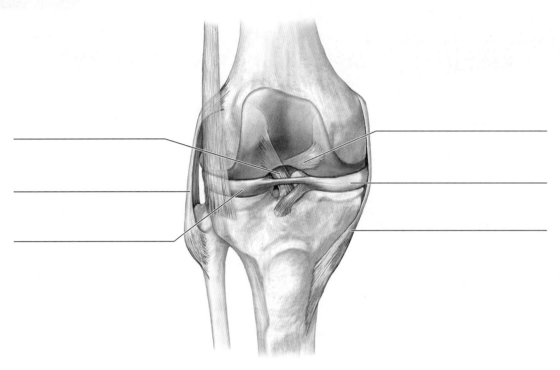

Figure 7.44

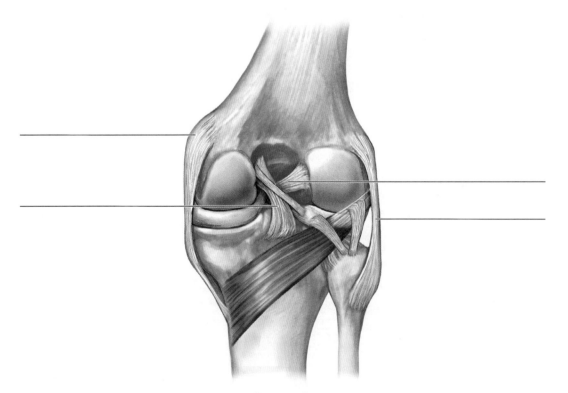

Figure 7.45

The Ankle

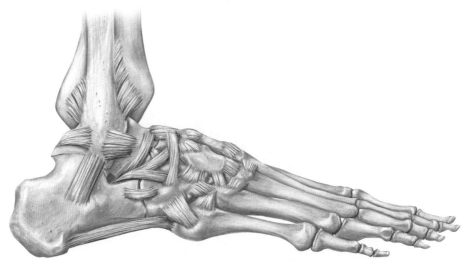

Figure 7.46 Lateral view of foot, bones and ligaments

Study Questions

1. Name the bones that articulate to form the ankle joint.

   _____

   _____

2. Name and explain specifically the four movements allowed at the ankle joint.

   _____

   _____

3. While jogging, your foot fell into a pothole resulting in a sore ankle. The doctor
   determined that you "sprained your ankle." Describe what a sprain is.

   _____

   _____

Joints of the Vertebral Column

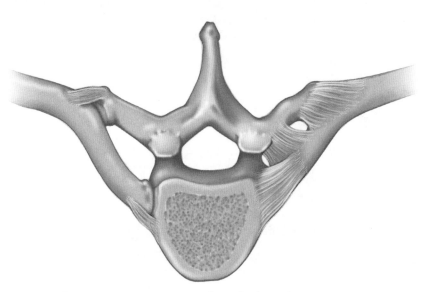

Figure 7.47 Superior view of vertebral attachment to ribs

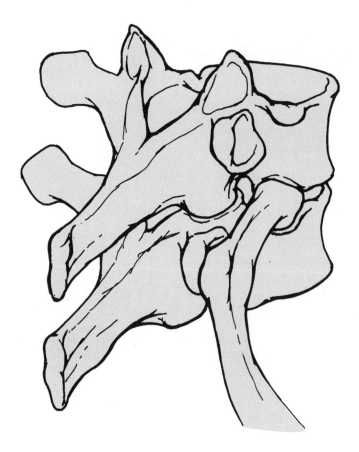

Figure 7.48 Vertebrae, posterior view

Study Questions

1. What type of joint is located between the bodies of adjacent vertebrae (synarthrotic, amphiarthrotic, diarthrotic)?

   _____

   _____

2. Name the processes that articulate to form a "zygapophyseal" joint between any adjacent vertebrae.

   _____

   _____

3. What type of synovial joint is a "zygapophyseal" joint (saddle, hinge, pivot, ball and socket, condyloid, gliding)?

   _____

   _____

4. Name the joint formed between the occipital bone and the first cervical vertebra (atlas) and describe which movements of the skull can be performed because of the presence of this joint.

   _____

   _____

5. Name the joint formed between C1 (atlas) and C2 (axis) and describe which movements of the skull can be performed because of the existence of this joint.

   _____

   _____

The Muscular System

Objectives

After completing this laboratory exercise, students will be able to:

1. Identify skeletal muscles in each region of the body.
2. Define the concept of origin and insertion in relation to skeletal muscle anatomy.
3. Describe the process of excitation/contraction coupling in skeletal muscle contraction.
4. Identify the phases of a skeletal muscle twitch.
5. Demonstrate a single twitch, summation, tetanus, and fatigue in skeletal muscle.

Overview

The purpose of this laboratory exercise is to familiarize you with the anatomical location of representative skeletal muscles from each region of the body. Once you are familiar with the major muscle groups, you will be introduced to the concept of origin/insertion of skeletal muscles. You will then tie the foundational anatomical knowledge you just learned and demonstrate the contractile mechanism of skeletal muscles.

Lab Materials

- Models that show muscles of the head and the neck, trunk, upper limb, and upper limb. (Preserved or plastinated cadavers with proper dissections may be substituted.)
  - ☐ Grip strength and electromyogram (iWorx exercise HM-1)
- ☐ http://www.iworx.com/home/
- ☐ http://www.iworx.com/LabExercises/ lockedexercises/LockedEMG-GripStrength-LS2.pdf
- ☐ PC Computer
- ☐ IWX/214 data acquisition unit
- ☐ USB cable
- ☐ IWX/214 power supply
- ☐ C-AAMI-504 ECG cable and electrode lead wires
- ☐ Disposable electrodes
- ☐ FT-325 hand dynamometer
- ☐ Alcohol swabs
- ☐ Bathroom scale and five or six textbooks
- ☐ String
- ☐ Metric ruler

Exercises

Exercise 8.1: Skeletal muscle anatomy
  8.1-1: Muscles of the head and the neck
  8.1-2: Muscles of the trunk
  8.1-3: Muscles of the upper limb
  8.1-4: Muscles of the lower limb
Exercise 8.2: Skeletal muscle contraction
  8.2-1: Grip strength and electromyogram (EMG) activity (using iWorx 214 and LabScribe V .20)
  8.2-2: EMG intensity and force in dominant arm

Exercise 8.2 is an optional exercise based on using iWorx physiological recording system.

Estimated lab time: 90 minutes

Instructions: For Exercises 8.1-1 to 8.1-4, use models (or cadavers) and refer to your textbook to help you find and label the indicated muscles in the figures provided.

Muscles of the Head and the Neck

Instructions: Label the following muscles in Figure 8.1:

- ■ Muscles of facial expression
  - ☐ Occipitofrontalis (frontal belly)
  - ☐ Orbicularis oculi
  - ☐ Orbicularis oris
- ■ Muscles of mastication
  - ☐ Masseter
  - ☐ Temporalis
- ■ Muscle to move the head
  - ☐ Sternocleidomastoid

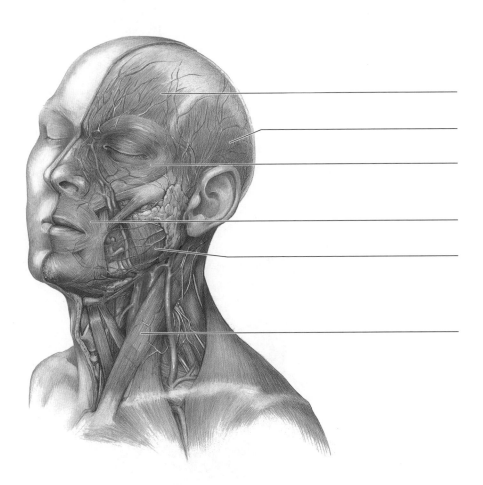

Figure 8.1

Muscles of the Trunk

Instructions: Label the following muscles in Figures 8.2 and 8.3:

- ■ Erector spinae group
- ■ Rectus abdominus
- ■ Transversus abdominus

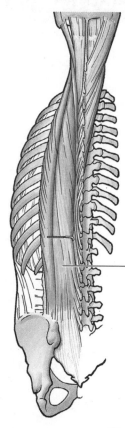

Figure 8.2

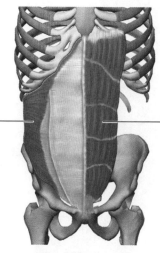

Figure 8.3

Muscles of the Upper Limb

Instructions: Label the following muscles in Figures 8.4 and 8.5:

- Muscles that position the pectoral girdle
  - ☐ Pectoralis minor
  - ☐ Serratus anterior
  - ☐ Levator scapulae
  - ☐ Rhomboid major
  - ☐ Rhomboid minor
  - ☐ Trapezius

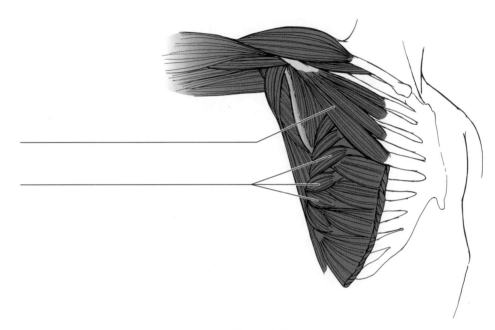

Figure 8.4

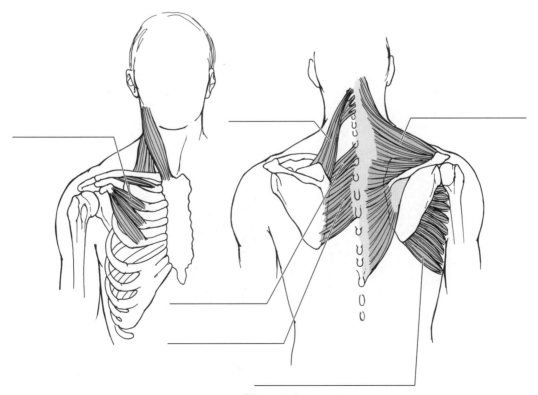

Figure 8.5

Instructions: Label the following muscles in Figures 8.6 and 8.7:

- Muscles that move the arm at the shoulder joint
    - ☐ Latissimus dorsi
    - ☐ Pectoralis major
    - ☐ Deltoid
- Muscles of the rotator cuff
    - ☐ Subscapularis
    - ☐ Infraspinatus
    - ☐ Teres minor

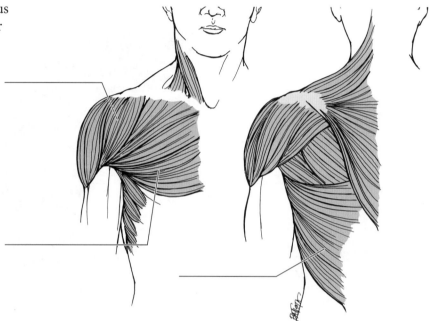

Figure 8.6

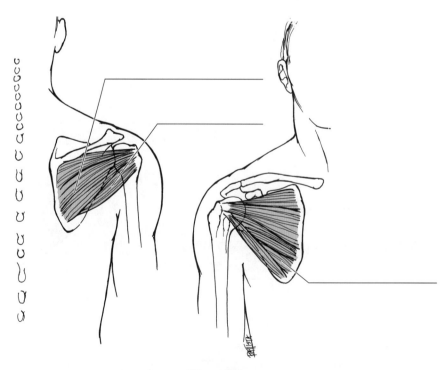

Figure 8.7

Instructions: Label the following muscles in Figure 8.8:

- ■ Muscles that move the forearm at the elbow joint
  - ☐ Biceps brachii
  - ☐ Brachialis
  - ☐ Brachioradialis
  - ☐ Triceps brachii
  - ☐ Pronator teres

- ■ Muscles that move the hand at the wrist joint
  - ☐ Anterior forearm (flexors)
    - ☐ Flexor carpi radialis
    - ☐ Flexor carpi ulnaris
    - ☐ Palmaris longus
  - ☐ Posterior forearm (extensors)
    - ☐ Extensor carpi radialis brevis
    - ☐ Extensor carpi radialis longus

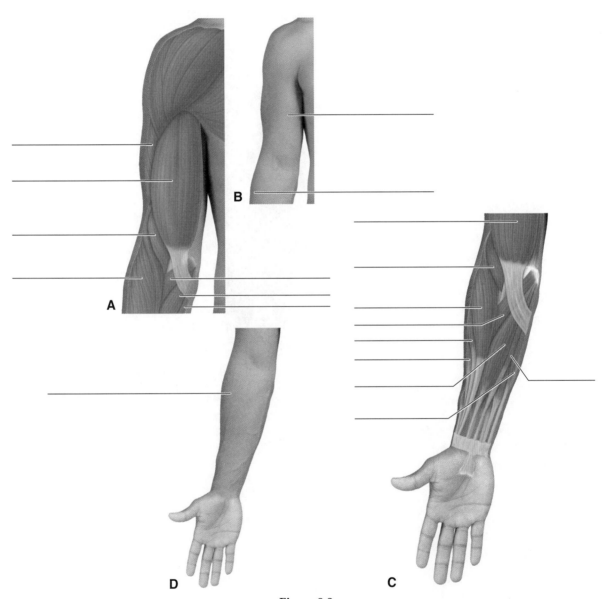

Figure 8.8

Exercise 8.1-4 | Muscles of the Lower Limb

Instructions: Label the following muscles in Figure 8.9:

■ Muscles that move the thigh at the hip joint
 ☐ Adductor longus
 ☐ Gracilis

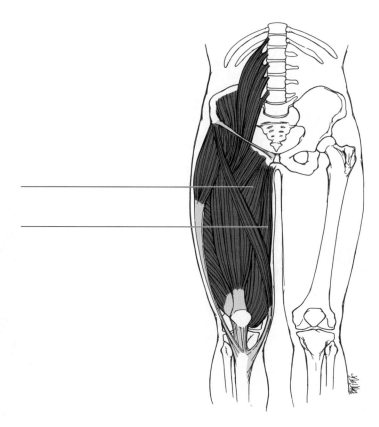

Figure 8.9

Instructions: Label the following muscles in Figure 8.10:

- Gluteus maximus
- Gluteus medius
- Gluteus minimus

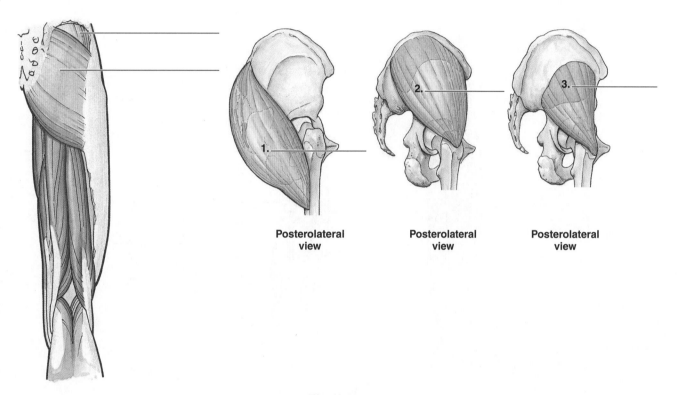

Posterolateral view

Posterolateral view

Posterolateral view

Figure 8.10

Instructions: Label the following muscles in Figures 8.11 and 8.12:

- ■ Muscles that move the leg at the knee joint
  - ☐ Quadriceps femoris
    - ☐ Rectus femoris
    - ☐ Vastus lateralis
    - ☐ Vastus medialis
  - ☐ Hamstrings
    - ☐ Biceps femoris
    - ☐ Semitendinosus
    - ☐ Semimembranosus

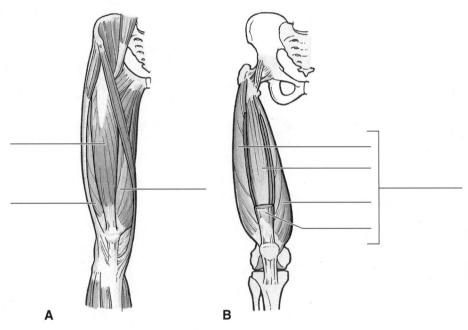

A   **B**

Figure 8.11

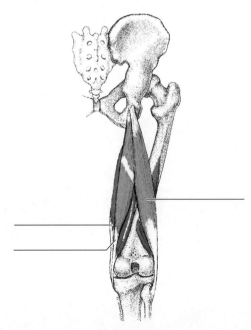

Figure 8.12

Instructions: Label the following muscles in Figures 8.13 and 8.14:

■ Muscles that move the foot and toes
- ☐ Tibialis anterior
- ☐ Gastrocnemius
- ☐ Soleus
- ☐ Fibularis (peroneus) longus
- ☐ Fibularis (peroneus) brevis

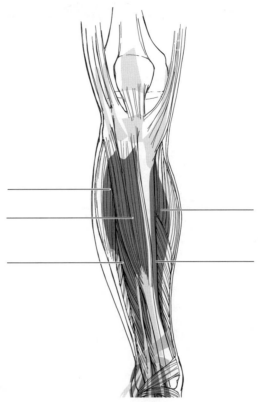

Figure 8.13

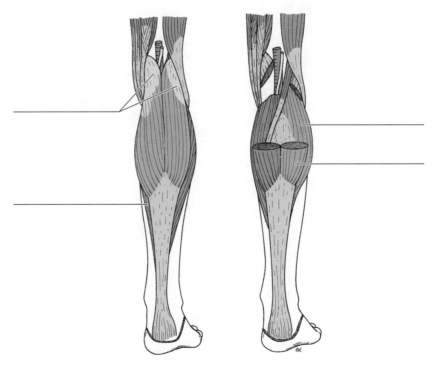

Figure 8.14

Skeletal Muscle Contraction

Exercise 8.2

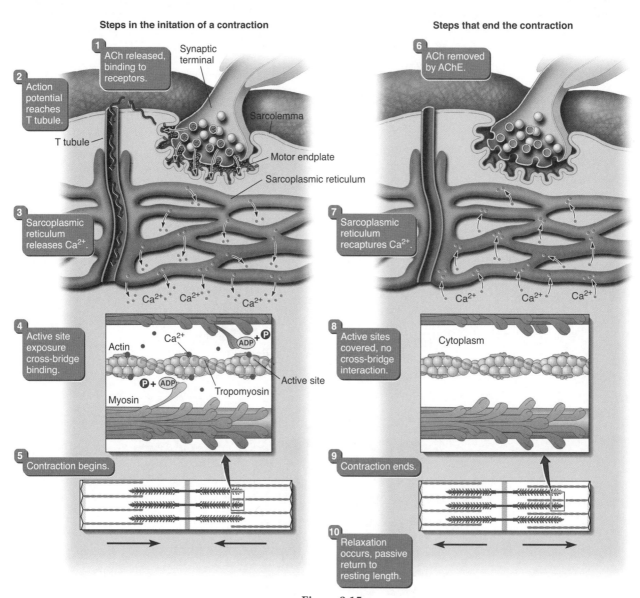

Figure 8.15

Skeletal muscle contraction is a fundamental process. Refer to your textbook for a detailed explanation. For this lab, refer to Figure 8.15.

Grip Strength and Electromyogram (EMG) Activity (Using iWorx 214 and LabScribe V .20)*

Optional Exercise 8.2-1

A motor unit is composed of a motor neuron and all the muscle fibers that are innervated by that motor neuron. In a persistent muscle contraction, multiple motor units fire repetitively throughout the contraction of the muscle. The strength of a muscle contraction is related to the number of motor units in the muscle that are activated during the same period. The EMG recorded during the muscle contraction is seen as a burst of spikelike signals, and the duration of the burst is approximately equal to the duration of the muscle contraction.

The strength of a striated muscle contraction is directly proportional to the amount of electrical activity in the muscle. However, it is difficult to quantify the amount of electrical activity in a muscle unless the raw EMG data are mathematically transformed. One of the most common transformations used is the integration of the absolute values of the amplitudes of the EMG spikes. Through this transformation, it has been found that the area under the graph of the absolute integral of the EMG is linearly proportional to the strength of the muscle contraction.

In this experiment, students will use a hand dynamometer to measure a subject's grip strength as the EMG activity of the forearm muscles used to generate the subject's grip is recorded. The EMG activity will be related to the grip strength by plotting the maximum grip strength as a function of the area under the absolute integral of the EMG activity during the muscle contraction. Data recordings will be made from the subject's dominant and nondominant forearms, and the relative strength and electrical activity of each forearm will be compared to its diameter. Recordings of prolonged grip strength and forearm EMG activity will also be made to determine the rate of fatigue in the dominant and nondominant forearms.

Instructions:

IWX/214 setup

1. Place the IWX/214 on the bench, close to the computer.

2. Use the USB cable to connect the computer to the USB port on the rear panel of the IWX/214.

3. Plug the power supply for the IWX/214 into the electrical outlet. Insert the plug on the end of the power supply cable into the labeled socket on the rear of the IWX/214. Use the power switch to turn on the unit. Confirm that the red power light is on.

Instructions:

Start the software

1. Click on the LabScribe shortcut on the computer's desktop to open the program. If a shortcut is not available, click on the Windows **Start menu** and move the cursor to **All Programs** and then to the listing for **iWorx**. Select **LabScribe** from the **iWorx submenu**. The LabScribe **Main window** will appear as the program opens.

2. On the **Main window**, pull down the **Settings menu** and select **Load Group**.

3. Locate the folder that contains the settings group, **IPLMv4.iwxgrp**. Select this group and click **Open**.

---

*Exercise reprinted with permission from iWorx: http://www.iworx.com/ LabExercises/lockedexercises/LockedEMG-GripStrength-LS2.pdf.

4. Pull down the **Settings menu** again. Select the **EMG-GripStrength-LS2** settings file.

5. After a short time, LabScribe will appear on the computer screen as configured by the **EMG-GripStrength-LS2** settings.

Instructions:

EMG cable and hand dynamometer setup

1. Locate the C-AAMI-504 EMG cable and electrode lead wires, and FT-325 hand dynamometer.

2. Plug the DIN8 connector to the FT-325 hand dynamometer into the Channel 3 input of the IWX/214.

3. Insert the black AAMI connector on the end of the EMG cable into the isolated inputs of Channels 1 and 2 of the IWX/214.

4. Insert the connectors on the red, black, and green electrode lead wires into the matching sockets on the lead pedestal of the EMG cable.

5. The subject should remove all jewelry from his or her wrists. For the first exercises in this lab, record EMGs and muscle forces from the subject's dominant arm, the arm used most often.

6. Use an alcohol swab to clean and scrub three regions on the inside of the subject's dominant forearm where the electrodes will be placed. One area is near the wrist, the second is in the middle of the forearm, and the third area is about 2 inches from the elbow.

7. Let the areas dry before attaching the electrodes.

8. Remove the plastic disk from a disposable electrode and apply it to one of the scrubbed areas. Repeat for the other two areas.

9. Snap the lead wires onto the electrodes so that
   a. the red "+1" lead is attached to the electrode near the elbow,
   b. the black "−1" lead is attached to the electrode in the middle of the forearm, and
   c. the green "C" lead (the ground) is attached to the electrode on the wrist.

Instructions:

Calibrating the hand dynamometer

1. Collect five textbooks. Weigh the stack of books on the bathroom scale. Record the weight of the stack in kilograms (kg). **Note:** Remember that 1 kg is equal to 2.2 pounds.

2. Lay the hand dynamometer down on the bench top. Click the **Record** button on the LabScribe **Main** window and record for 10 seconds.

3. Continue to record as you stack the textbooks on the bulb of the hand dynamometer. Record for an additional 10 seconds after the last book is placed on the stack. Click the **Stop** button.

4. Click the **AutoScale** button on the **Muscle Force** channel. Use the **Double Display Time** icon to adjust the **Display Time** of the **Main window** to display the force recording before and after the books were placed on the hand dynamometer.

5. Click on the **Double Cursors button** on the LabScribe toolbar. Place one cursor on the force recording made before the books were placed on the bulb. Place the other cursor on the recording after the books were placed on the bulb.

6. Open the **Channel Menu** of the **Muscle Force** channel by clicking on the **down arrow** to the left of the channels' title. Select **Units** from this menu and **Simple** from the submenu to open the **Simple Units Conversion dialogue window**.

7. Put check marks in the boxes next to **Apply Units to new data** and **Apply Units to all blocks**. Click on the **Units Off button** to remove any prior units conversion from this channel.

8. In the middle of the window is an array of four boxes. For each cursor, the value in the box on the left is the voltage at the position of the cursor on the recording window. In the box on the right, enter the value of the unit that equals the voltage on the left:
   a. For Cursor 1, type **zero (0)** in the box on the right. This cursor is on the portion of the recording when no weight was placed on top of the hand dynamometer.
   b. For Cursor 2, type the weight of the stack of books in the box on the right.
   c. Type the name of the unit, **kilogram** or **kg**, in the **Unit Name** box. Click the **OK** button.

EMG Intensity and Force in Dominant Arm*   Exercise 8.2-2

Aim: To determine the relationship between the intensity of EMG activity and the force of a muscle contraction in the subject's dominant arm.

Instructions:

Procedure

1. The subject should sit quietly with his or her dominant forearm resting on the table top. Explain the procedure to the subject. The subject will squeeze his or her fist around the hand dynamometer four times; each contraction is 2 seconds long followed by 2 seconds of relaxation. Each successive contraction should be approximately two, three, and four times stronger than the first contraction.

2. **Type Increasing Grip Force-Dominant** in the **Mark box** to the right of the **Mark button**. Click the **Record button** to begin the recording; then, press the **Enter** key on the keyboard to mark the beginning of the recording. After the recording is marked, tell the subject to begin squeezing the hand dynamometer following the procedure outlined in the step above.

3. In the relaxation period after the last contraction, click the **Stop** button.

4. Click the **AutoScale buttons** for the **EMG**, **Muscle Force**, and **EMG Integral** channels.

5. Select **Save As** in the **File menu** and type a name for the file. Choose a destination on the computer in which to save the file, like your lab group folder. Designate the file type as ***.iwxdata**. Click on the **Save** button to save the data file.

Instructions:

Data analysis

1. Use the **Display Time** icons to adjust the **Display Time** of the **Main window** to show the four progressive muscle contractions on the **Main window**. The four contractions can also

---

*Exercise reprinted with permission from iWorx: http://www.iworx.com/ LabExercises/lockedexercises/LockedEMG-GripStrength-LS2.pdf.

be selected by placing the cursors on either side of a group of four contractions, clicking the **Zoom between Cursors** button on the LabScribe toolbar to expand the segment with the four contractions to the width of the **Main window**.

2. Click on the **Analysis window** icon in the toolbar or select **Analysis** from the **Windows menu** to transfer the data displayed in the **Main window** to the **Analysis window**.

3. Look at the **Function Table** that is above the uppermost channel displayed in the **Analysis window**. The mathematical functions, **Abs. Area**, **V2-V1**, and **T2-T1**, should appear in this table. The values for **Abs. Area**, **V2-V1**, and **T2-T1** on each channel are seen in the table across the top margin of each channel.

4. Use the mouse to click on and drag the cursors to the beginning and end of the first muscle contraction. The values for **Abs. Area** on the **EMG** and **Muscle channels** are the relative amount of the electrical activity causing the contraction and relative strength of the muscle, respectively. Record the values.

5. Repeat steps 2, 3, and 4 for the other three muscle contractions recorded in this exercise.

Study Questions

1. Plot the absolute area of muscle contraction as a function of the absolute area of the EMG signals for each muscle clinch.

2. Is there a linear relationship between the absolute area under EMG signals and the absolute area under the muscle contraction?

   _____

   _____

   _____

3. Do muscle fibers have a refractory period like nerve fibers?

   _____

   _____

   _____

4. Does the amplitude of the EMG signal and the force of contraction, as measured by the absolute areas, increase because a finite number of fibers fire more often or because more fibers are employed to fire as the intensity of signals in the motor neurons increases, or a combination of these two?

   _____

   _____

   _____

The Nervous System

Objectives

After completing this laboratory exercise, students will be able to:

1. Identify the name, number, and function of the 12 pairs of cranial nerves.
2. Perform a separate functional test of each cranial nerve.
3. Identify major structures in the brain.
4. Identify major structures in the spinal cord.
5. Elicit deep-tendon, superficial, and cutaneous reflexes.

Overview

In this laboratory exercise, you will be exposed to the basic anatomy of the central nervous system. You and your lab partner will perform several exercises to demonstrate cranial nerve function. Each of these exercises is a simple example of the various tests that may take place in a neurologist's office. If the test turns out as expected, for example, you can smell properly, there is no neurological defect in a particular area. If on the other hand, a particular test is negative, it gives the clinician a window into the possible cause of the dysfunction.

Apply this exercise to gain an appreciation for the flow of information from the environment into the brain, and then use your brain to understand and react to the incoming information.

Lab Materials

- Brain and spinal cord models
- Small flashlights
- Two types of cola or soda
- Rubber hammers
- Two-point discrimination caliper (Carolina Biological)
- Unlabeled smell samples (common household materials in unlabeled bottles)
- Blind spot test cards
- Color blindness test charts
- 3D stereogram pictures
- Retractable ink pens (or similar device for making clicking noise)
- Swivel chair
- Tuning forks
- Tongue depressors
- Long-handle cotton swabs

Exercises

Exercise 9.1: Anatomy of the brain
Exercise 9.2: Anatomy of the spinal cord
Exercise 9.3: The cranial nerves
  9.3-1: Cranial nerve I, the olfactory nerve
  9.3-2: Cranial nerve II, the optic nerve
  9.3-3: Cranial nerve III, the oculomotor nerve
  9.3-4: Cranial nerve IV, the trochlear nerve and cranial nerve VI, the abducens nerve
  9.3-5: Cranial nerve V, the trigeminal nerve
  9.3-6: Cranial nerve VII, the facial nerve
  9.3-7: Cranial nerve VIII, the vestibulocochlear nerve
  9.3-8: Cranial nerve IX, the glossopharyngeal nerve
  9.3-9: Cranial nerve X, the vagus nerve
  9.3-10: Cranial nerve XI, the spinal accessory nerve
  9.3-11: Cranial nerve XII, the hypoglossal nerve
  9.3-12: Names of the cranial nerves and their function
Exercise 9.4: The reflex arc

Estimated lab time: 90 minutes

Anatomy of the Brain

Instructions: Refer to your textbook and use the models provided in your lab to observe the following structures. As you find them on the models, label them in Figures 9.1 to 9.3.

- Frontal, parietal, occipital, and temporal lobes
- Corpus collusum
- Thalamus
- Pituitary gland
- Pons
- Medulla
- Cerebellum
- Lateral ventricle
- Gyrus
- Sulci

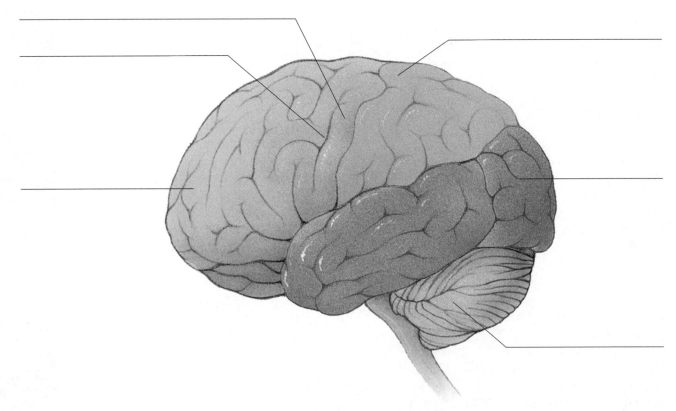

Figure 9.1

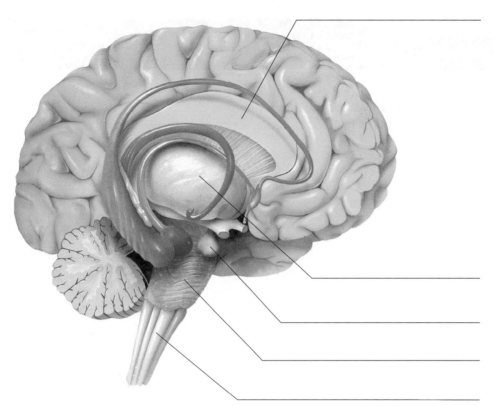

Figure 9.2

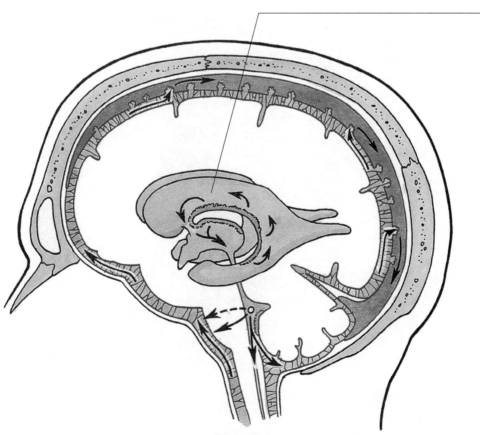

Figure 9.3

Anatomy of the Spinal Cord

Instructions: Refer to your textbook and use the models provided in your lab to observe the following structures found in the spinal cord and label them in Figures 9.4 and 9.5.

- Dura mater
- Pia mater
- Arachnoid mater
- Dorsal root ganglion
- Ventral root
- Spinal nerve

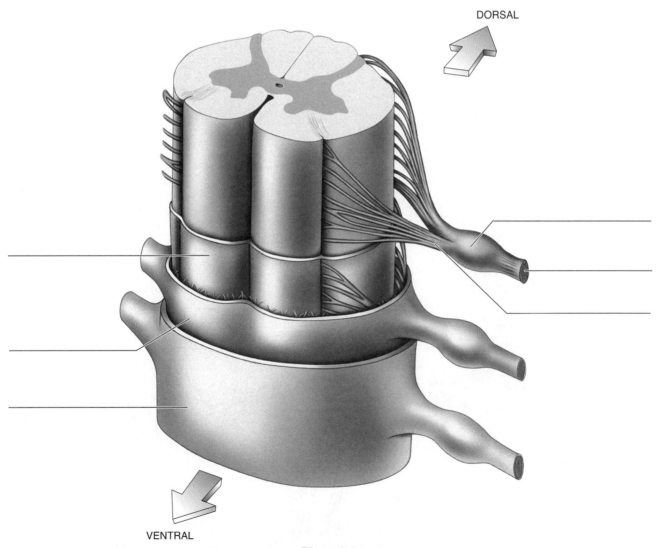

DORSAL

VENTRAL

Figure 9.4

■ Spinal cord
■ Spinal nerves
■ Conus medullaris
■ Cauda equina

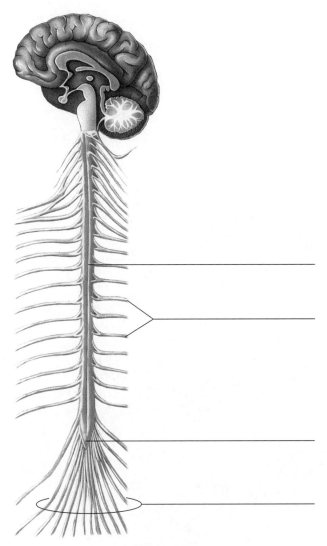

Figure 9.5

The Cranial Nerves

Instructions: Refer to your textbook and use the models provided in your lab to perform the following exercises to demonstrate the function of each cranial nerve. At the end of the exercise, you will come to know the name, number, function, and a basic test for each cranial nerve.

Inferior view

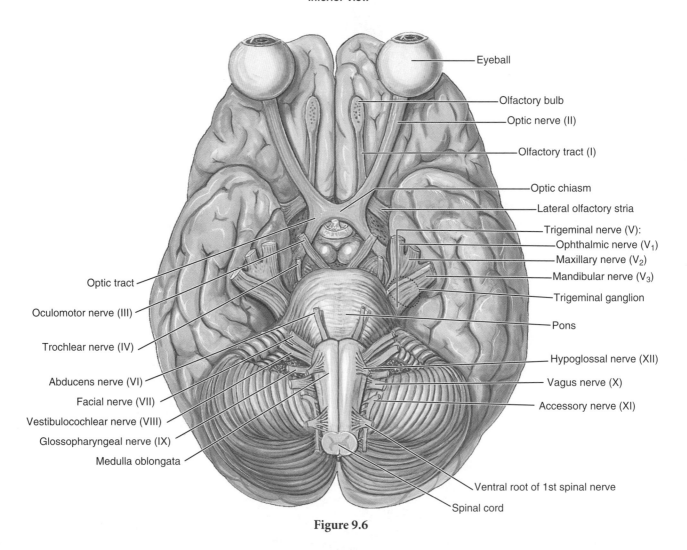

Figure 9.6

Cranial Nerve I, the Olfactory Nerve

Instructions: This nerve provides the sense of smell. To test the function of this nerve, perform the following tasks:

1. Have your lab partner close his or her eyes.

2. Waft a series of different substances under your lab partner's nose.

3. Ask him or her to identify the smell.

Cranial Nerve II, the Optic Nerve

Instructions: This nerve provides the sense of sight. To test the functionality of the optic nerve, perform the following tasks:

1. Read the time off the clock with both eyes and then with only one eye at a time.

2. Close your eyes and gently press on the sides of your eyes. What do you see?

   _____

   _____

   _____

3. Blind spot test

   a. Hold the card at arm's length, straight out from your nose.

   b. Close your left eye and focus on the circle (not the X).

   c. Slowly pull the card toward you until the X disappears. You have found your blind spot. Now explain why you have a blind spot and why you do not notice it.

   _____

   _____

   _____

4. Test for color blindness

   a. Read the four numbers in the color test plates

Cranial Nerve III, the Oculomotor Nerve

Cranial nerve III has many functions.

1. Controls movement of the eyeball. What is the purpose of this?

   _____

   _____

   _____

2. Controls size of the pupil. What is the purpose of this?

   _____

   _____

   _____

3. Controls shape of the lens. What is the purpose of this?

_____

_____

_____

Instructions: To test the functionality of the oculomotor nerve, perform the following tasks:

1. Have your lab partner follow your finger with his or her eyes as you move it up and down and then side to side.

2. Shine a penlight into your lab partner's eye and observe constriction of the pupil in that same eye (**direct light reflex**) and constriction of the opposite pupil (**consensual light reflex**).

3. Test your lab partner's ability to focus (**accommodation**) by having him or her stare at the Magic Eye pictures until the 3D object appears.

Exercise 9.3-4 — Cranial Nerve IV, the Trochlear Nerve and Cranial Nerve VI, the Abducens Nerve

Cranial nerves IV and VI innervate the muscles that move the eyeball and are usually examined together.

Instructions: To examine the functionality of these cranial nerves, perform the following tests:

1. Hold an index finger approximately 1 ft in front of your lab partner's face. Instruct your lab partner to follow your finger as you do the following:
   a. Up and down—test for cranial nerve III
   b. Left and right—test for cranial nerve VI
   c. Diagonally—test for cranial nerve IV

Exercise 9.3-5 — Cranial Nerve V, the Trigeminal Nerve

The trigeminal nerve has mixed functions, as it has both sensory and motor functions. It provides sensation to the skin of the forehead, cheeks, lower jaw, teeth, and gums, and innervates the skeletal muscles involved in mastication.

Instructions: To test the sensory component of this nerve, perform the following tasks:

1. Instruct your lab partner to close his or her eyes.

2. Poke the skin of your lab partner's forehead, cheek, and mandible with your finger.

3. Have your lab partner indicate when the touch sensation is felt by saying "now."

   To test the motor function of the trigeminal nerve, perform the following tasks:

1. Instruct your lab partner to open and close his or her jaw.

2. Instruct your lab partner to move the jaw from side to side.

Cranial Nerve VII, the Facial Nerve

Exercise 9.3-6

The facial nerve also has mixed functions, as it has both sensory and motor functions. It provides the sense of taste and innervates the muscles of facial expression.

Instructions: To test the sensory portion of this nerve, perform the following tasks:

1. With his or her eyes closed, ask your lab partner to take a sip of either Coke or Pepsi, without telling him or her which one you are supplying.

2. After a few minutes, give your lab partner a sip of the opposite beverage from the one used in step 1.

3. Ask your lab partner to identify each beverage.

   To test the motor portion of this nerve, observe your lab partner as he or she performs the following actions:

- Pucker the lips
- Wink
- Puff the cheeks
- Smile
- Wiggle the ears

Cranial Nerve VIII, the Vestibulocochlear Nerve

Exercise 9.3-7

This nerve provides the sense of hearing, balance, and equilibrium.

Instructions: To test the hearing function of this nerve, perform the following tasks:

1. Stand behind your seated lab partner, holding pens next to his or her ears.

2. With your lab partner's eyes closed, click either the left or right pen.

3. Ask your lab partner which pen is being clicked.

   To test the sense of balance and equilibrium, perform the following tasks:

1. Spin your lab partner several rotations in a swivel chair.

2. Stop the chair and immediately observe oscillations of the eyeball (nystagmus).

Cranial Nerve IX, the Glossopharyngeal Nerve

Exercise 9.3-8

This nerve provides the sense of taste to the back portion of the tongue, sensory to the pharyngeal walls, and innervates the muscles of the pharynx (throat).

Instructions: To test the function of this nerve, perform the gag reflex:

1. While depressing the tongue with a depressor, lightly touch the side walls of the patient's throat with a cotton-tipped applicator.

2. Observe the movement of the uvula (soft palate). *Warning:* Do not stand directly in front of your partner.

3. Next time you get a sore throat, appreciate the existence of this nerve.

Cranial Nerve X, the Vagus Nerve

Exercise 9.3-9

The vagus nerve innervates skeletal muscles used in swallowing and muscles of the vocal cords. In addition, the vagus nerve innervates visceral organs (heart, stomach, intestines). Usually, cranial nerves IX and X are tested simultaneously, but tests for the vagus nerve include deviation of the uvula to one side of the pharynx, hoarseness in the voice, and difficulty in swallowing.

Instructions: Perform this simple test for functionality of the vagus nerve:

1. Hold your hand over your throat and swallow.

2. Palpate (feel) the movements of structures in your throat.

3. Observe the uvula for any deviations.

Cranial Nerve XI, the Spinal Accessory Nerve

Exercise 9.3-10

This nerve innervates the muscles of the neck that move the head (sternocleidomastoid and trapezius).

Instructions: To test the function of this nerve, perform the following tasks:

1. Apply slight pressure to the side of your lab partner's head.

2. Instruct your lab partner to push against the resistance.

3. Repeat this process to the opposite side of the head.

4. Push your lab partner's head forward and ask him or her to resist the force.

5. Apply pressure to your lab partner's shoulder while he or she is seated and ask him or her to try to shrug his or her shoulders.

Cranial Nerve XII, the Hypoglossal Nerve

This nerve innervates the muscles of the tongue.

Instructions: To test the function of this nerve, perform the following tasks:

1. Instruct your lab partner to stick the tongue straight out.

2. Observe the movement and check for any deviations to the left or the right.

3. Now, instruct your lab partner to move the tongue to the left and then to the right.

4. Now, tell your lab partner to retract the tongue and close the mouth.

Names of the Cranial Nerves and their Function

Write specifically the names of the cranial nerves and their functions

	Name of Cranial Nerve	Function of Cranial Nerve
I		
II		
III		
IV		
V		Sensory: Motor:
VI		
VII		Sensory: Motor:
VIII		
IX		
X		
XI		
XII		

Exercise 9.4   The Reflex Arc

One of the most common and simplest tasks of the nervous system is the muscular reflex.

Instructions: Refer to Figure 9.7 to familiarize yourself with the reflex arc and label the following elements in it:

- Effector organ
- Interneuron
- Motor neuron
- Peripheral receptor
- Sensory neuron

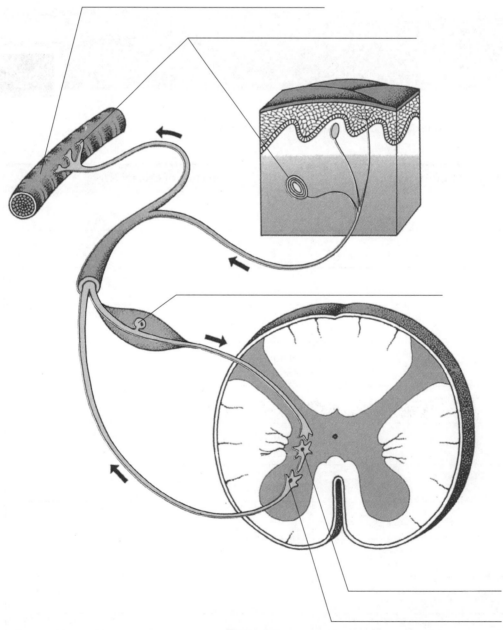

Figure 9.7

The knee-jerk, or patellar tendon reflex is an example of a stretch reflex. This reflex is also called a "deep-tendon reflex." To test for the functional integrity of all the components of a simple, deep-tendon reflex, have your lab partner sit on a table with his or her legs dangling freely over the edge. Use a rubber mallet to swiftly tap the patellar tendon below the patella. As the tendon (and quadriceps muscle) stretches, the nervous system monitors this change in length and, reflexively, resists this change by stimulating the quadriceps muscle to contract. Contraction of the muscle causes it to shorten (and, thus, restores its original length) and also produces extension of the leg.

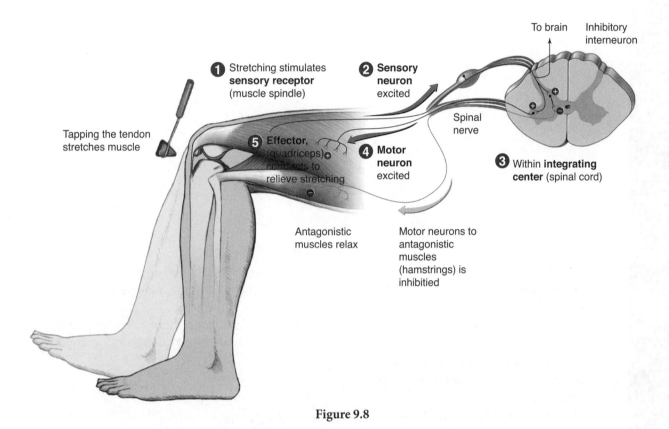

Figure 9.8

If your lab partner is resistant to this reflex, have him or her press his or her palms together very tightly. While he or she is performing this maneuver, repeat the test for the knee-jerk reflex. This is referred to as the Jendrassik method of reinforcement.

The Cardiovascular System

Objectives

After completing this laboratory exercise, students will be able to:

1. Determine heart rate, pulse rate, respiratory rate, and blood pressure.
2. Analyze an electrocardiogram (EKG) and be able to label the waveforms as well as calculate heart rate.
3. Determine their own level of physical fitness.
4. Identify the major structures of the heart and the major vessels.

Overview

This lab exercise is designed to expose you to the basic anatomy and physiology of the cardiovascular system. By using the models and standard medical equipment, you will learn the fundamentals of the cardiovascular system.

Lab Materials

- Stethoscope
- Stopwatch
- EKG recorder
- Manual sphygmomanometer
- Automatic sphygmomanometer
- Models of the heart
- Histological preparations of cardiac muscle and arterial cross section showing smooth muscle
- Exercise bike

Exercises

Exercise 10.1: Determination of heart rate, pulse rate, respiratory rate, and blood pressure

Exercise 10.2: Determination of heart rate and labeling of waves from an electrocardiogram

Exercise 10.3: Determination of index of physical fitness

Exercise 10.4: Anatomy of the human heart

Estimated lab time: 90 minutes

Determination of Heart Rate, Pulse Rate, Respiratory Rate, and Blood Pressure

Exercise 10.1

Do not perform the experiment on yourself; you should measure the following events on another individual in your group. First complete each measurement with your subject at rest. Then have your subject exercise at a moderate pace for 5 minutes and repeat the measurements immediately following the exercise.

Instructions:

1. Heart rate: Use a stethoscope to listen for heart sounds. The sounds are paired, "lub-dub" for each beat, and correspond to the closing of valves in the heart. Count the beats for one full minute and record the rate in beats per minute.

   a. Heart rate at rest: _____

   b. Heart rate following exercise: _____

   c. Percentage change: _____

2. Pulse rate: Feel the radial pulse and count the beats for a full minute and record the rate in beats per minute.

   a. Pulse rate at rest: _____

   b. Pulse rate following exercise: _____

   c. Percentage change: _____

3. Respiratory rate: Count the number of breaths taken per minute, simply by watching for inflation and deflation of the chest.

   a. Respiratory rate at rest: _____

   b. Respiratory rate following exercise: _____

   c. Percentage change: _____

4. Measure blood pressure using the digital sphygmomanometer and record the pressure as systolic/diastolic.

   a. Blood pressure at rest: _____

   b. Blood pressure following exercise: _____

   c. Percentage change: _____

Study Questions

1. Did all of the above measures increase or decrease following exercise?

   _____

   _____

2. Propose a plausible explanation for why the above measures either increased or decreased.

   _____

   _____

Determination of Heart Rate and Labeling of Waves from an Electrocardiogram

Exercise 10.3

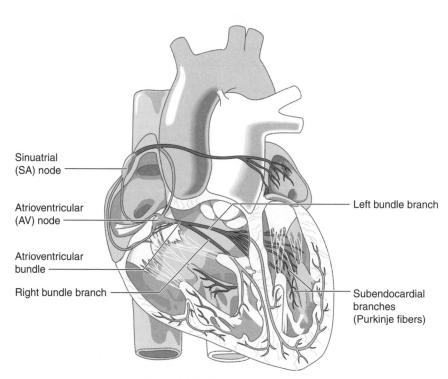

Figure 10.1 Heart, anterior view

Instructions: Describe the function of the following portions of the conducting system of the heart:

▪ SA node:

_____

_____

_____

▪ AV node:

_____

_____

_____

▪ Bundle branches:

_____

_____

_____

▪ Purkinje fibers:

_____

_____

_____

Instructions: In Figure 10.2, label the following components:

▪ P wave
▪ QRS complex
▪ T wave

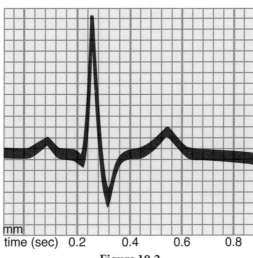

Figure 10.2

Instructions: Now explain the relationship of each peak to the contraction cycle of the heart:

■ P wave:

_____

_____

_____

■ QRS complex:

_____

_____

_____

■ T wave:

_____

_____

_____

Pick one member of the group and send him or her to the electrocardiogram (EKG) station, where the lab instructor will record his or her EKG for 1 to 2 minutes. Once the data are obtained, return to your seat for analysis.

Analysis of EKG Data

1. Pick one complete cycle and label the p wave, QRS complex, and the t wave.

2. Mark off a 15-second time frame on your data using the time event marks, remembering to start at 0. Count the number of complete heart cycles (one cycle is a p wave, a QRS complex, and a t wave) in your 15 seconds and use the calculation below to figure the heart rate.

$$HR = \frac{\#Beats}{seconds} \times \frac{60}{1\,minute}$$

Show your work here:

Determination of Index of Physical Fitness

Instructions: In this experiment, measure the radial pulse of your subject before and after exercise. Pay close attention to the time and measure for 15 seconds at each indicated interval. For the exercise, have the subject ride the exercise bike for 5 minutes at a moderate pace.

Record the number of pulses that occur in 15 seconds for each of the following conditions:

1. At rest (before exercise) = _____

2. Immediately after exercise = _____

3. 15 seconds after exercise = _____

4. 30 seconds after exercise = _____

5. 2 minutes after exercise = _____

   a. Total (sum) = _____

   b. Average = _____

Use the table below to find your fitness level.

Heart Rate	Fitness Rating
Pulse average over 157	Poor
133–157	Fair
108–132	Average
83–107	Good
Below 83	Excellent

Exercise 10.4 | Anatomy of the Human Heart

Instructions: Refer to your textbook and use the models of the human heart to identify the following structures and label them in Figures 10.3 to 10.5.

- Right atrium
- Right ventricle
- Left atrium
- Left ventricle
- Tricuspid valve
- Bicuspid valve
- Aortic semilunar valve
- Pulmonary semilunar valve
- Superior vena cava
- Aorta
- Pulmonary trunk
- Intraventricular septum
- Apex of heart
- Myocardium

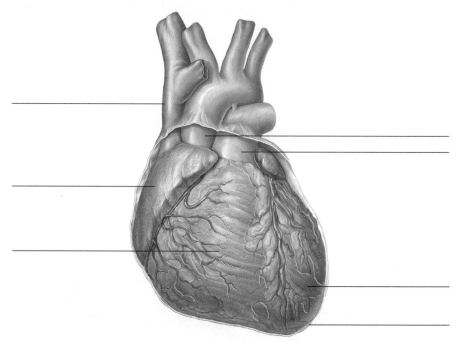

Figure 10.3

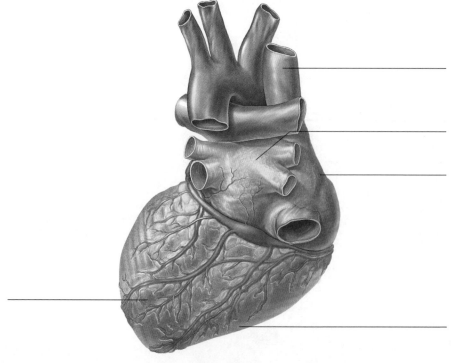

Figure 10.4

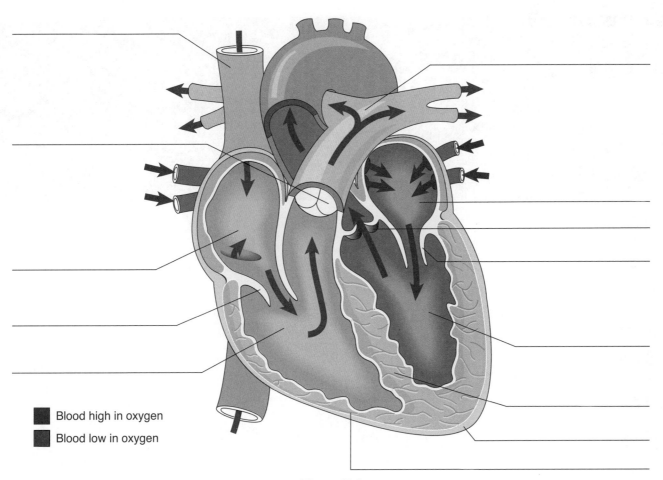

Blood high in oxygen

Blood low in oxygen

Figure 10.5

The Lymphatic System

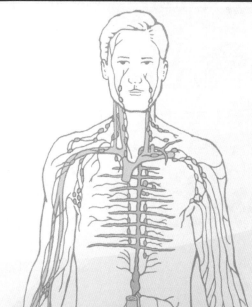

Objectives

After completing this laboratory exercise, students will be able to:

1. Describe the function of the lymphatic system.
2. Identify major lymphatic pathways and lymphatic organs.
3. Describe the structure of a lymph node.
4. Describe lymphatic fluid.
5. Explain lymphatic circulation.

Overview

The lymphatic system is composed of vessels that transport excess fluid from the tissues and interstitial spaces back to the circulatory system. In the process, the fluid is screened at specific nodes for foreign cells. When an invading organism is found, the general and specific immune responses are activated.

In this laboratory exercise, you will become familiar with the major vessels and specific structures of the lymphatic system. You will also be introduced to the general functions of the lymphatic tissue.

Lab Materials

- Models showing the major vessels and nodes of the lymphatic system
- Models showing lymphatic capillaries and lacteals
- Model of the spleen
- Microscopic slide of the splenic tissue
- Microscopic slide of the thymic tissue

Exercises

Exercise 11.1: Lymphatic vessels

Exercise 11.2: Structure of lymphatic vessels

Exercise 11.3: The spleen

Exercise 11.4: The lymphatic interaction with the immune system

Estimated lab time: 45 minutes

Lymphatic Vessels

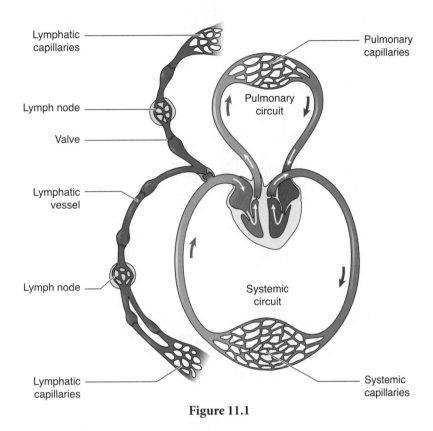

Figure 11.1

Instructions: In Figure 11.1, trace the flow of fluid from the circulatory system to the lymphatic system. After learning in your textbook that blood flow is driven by hydrostatic pressure, explain why fluid leaks from the capillaries into the interstitial space. Also, what would happen if we did not have a lymphatic system?

_____

_____

_____

_____

_____

_____

Exercise 11.2 | Structure of Lymphatic Vessels

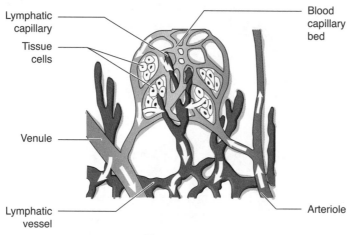

Lymphatic capillary
Tissue cells
Venule
Lymphatic vessel
Blood capillary bed
Arteriole

Figure 11.2

Figure 11.2 shows a typical lymphatic capillary. The lymphatic capillaries are closed-end tubes composed of a single layer of squamous epithelial cells. The single layer of cells is permeable to the interstitial fluid, allowing the interstitial fluid to drain into the vessel. From there, the fluid (now lymphatic fluid) moves into larger lymphatic vessels, then to lymph nodes, and finally to the lymphatic organs.

Instructions: Draw and describe the structure of a lymph capillary, a lymphatic vessel, and a lymph node. Be sure to include any special structures such as openings, valves, etc.

The Spleen

The spleen is an important lymphatic organ. It removes old fragile red blood cells (RBCs) and foreign particles from circulation. Located on the left side of the body, it sits adjacent to the stomach. It is highly vascular with a very large capillary network. This network facilitates the destruction of weak RBCs as they are forced through the capillary wall by hydrostatic pressure.

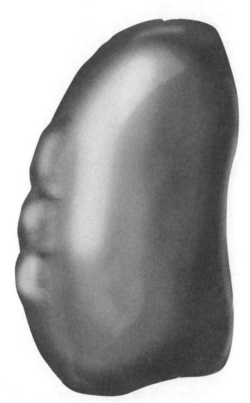

Figure 11.3

Instructions: In Figure 11.4, label the following structures:

■ Splenic artery
■ Splenic vein
■ Hilum

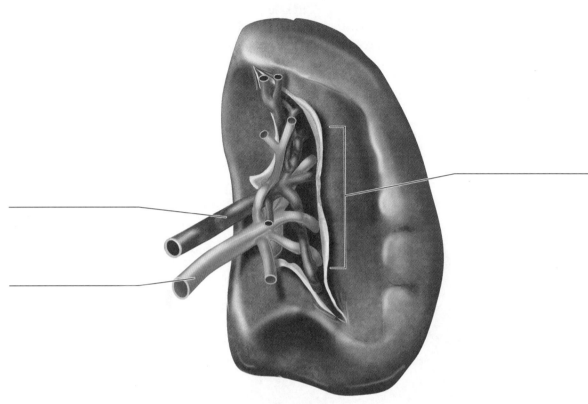

Figure 11.4

Instructions: Observe a microscopic preparation of splenic tissue. Identify the red pulp, white pulp, and an artery. Define the following:

1. White pulp:

_____

_____

_____

2. Red pulp:

_____

_____

_____

The Lymphatic Interaction With the Immune System

Exercise 11.4

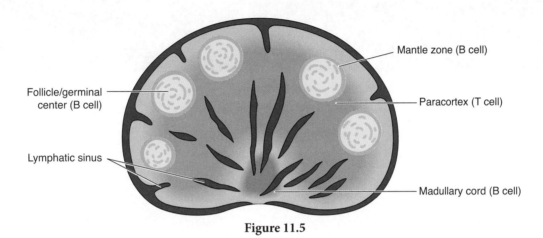

Figure 11.5

The primary immune cells are B cells and T cells.

Instructions: In basic terms, define the function of each cell.

1. B cell:

_____

_____

_____

2. T cell:

_____

_____

_____

   After learning in your textbook about the function and structure of the lymphatic system, explain why it makes sense for B and T cells to be found in the lymph nodes.

_____

_____

_____

_____

_____

_____

The Respiratory System

Objectives

After completing this laboratory exercise, students will be able to:

1. Operate two similar types of respirometers to measure various lung volumes.
2. Perform a pulmonary function test to determine the relative amount of airway resistance.
3. Perform a test to confirm that expired air is acidic due to the carbon dioxide gas.
4. Demonstrate how the levels of carbon dioxide stimulate the respiratory cycle.
5. List the muscles involved in breathing and explain the changes in air pressure associated with inhalation and exhalation.

Overview

The purpose of this lab exercise is to familiarize you with the basic anatomy and physiology of the pulmonary system as well as the respiratory cycle and associated anatomical structures. Each of the exercises is designed to demonstrate a fundamental concept of external respiration.

Lab Materials

- Phipps and Bird spirometer
- Harvard respirometer
- Disposable mouth pieces
- Recording paper
- Blow juice
    - ☐ 200 mL of water
    - ☐ 5 mL of 0.1 M NaOH (sodium hydroxide)
    - ☐ Three drops of phenolphthalein (color indicator for basic solution)
- Straws
- Six 200-mL beakers

Exercises

Exercise 12.1: Use of the Phipps and Bird spirometer to measure vital capacity

Exercise 12.2: Use of the Harvard spirometer to obtain various lung volumes

Exercise 12.3: Determination of airway resistance ($Fev_{1.0}/Fvc$)

Exercise 12.4: Acid test of expired air

Exercise 12.5: Effects of hyperventilation on breath holding

Exercise 12.6: The respiratory cycle

Estimated lab time: 90 minutes

Use of the Phipps and Bird Spirometer to Measure Vital Capacity

Exercise 12.1

Instructions: Follow the directions from your instructor on using the spirometer to record the vital capacity (VC) of five males and five females in the class and calculate their average value (in liters).

	Vital Capacity
Male 1	
Male 2	
Male 3	
Male 4	
Male 5	
Female 1	
Female 2	
Female 3	
Female 4	
Female 5	
Average	

Study Questions

1. Is there a difference between the average value for males and females?

   _____

   _____

2. What factor(s) might account for this difference?

   _____

   _____

   _____

Use of the Harvard Spirometer to Obtain Various Lung Volumes

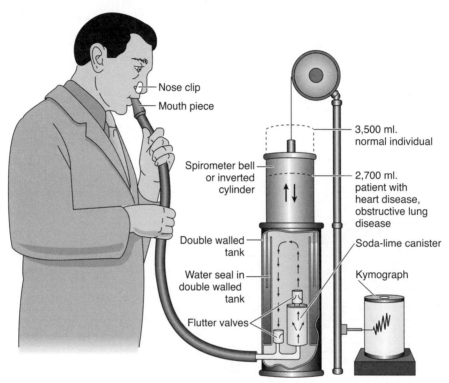

Figure 12.1 Spirometry.

Instructions: Choose one person to be the subject for your group. Allow the subject to adjust to breathing through the apparatus for about 15 seconds. Record resting tidal volumes (TVs) for 1 minute and calculate the respiratory rate for the subject. To obtain inspiratory reserve volume (IRV), inhale maximally, and to obtain the expiratory reserve volume (ERV), exhale maximally. To measure vital capacity, use the point of maximal inspiration to the point of maximal expiration.

Mark all measurements (in centimeters) and label all the lung volumes on the recording. Use the following conversion factor in your calculations of lung volumes:

$$VC = IRV + TV + ERV$$

Instructions: Calculate the following variables:

1. Tidal volume

2. Inspiratory reserve volume

3. Expiratory reserve volume

4. Vital capacity

5. Respiratory rate (breaths per minute)

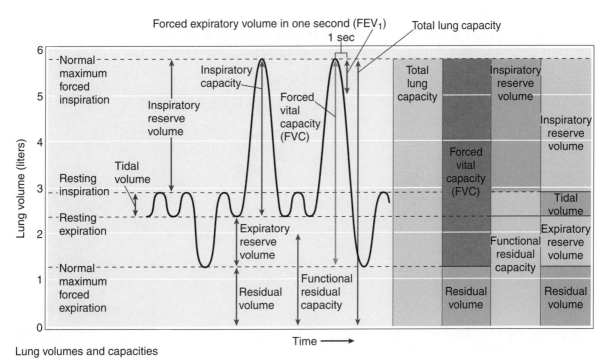

Figure 12.2 Lung capacities.

Determination of Airway Resistance ($Fev_{1.0}/Fvc$)

Exercise 12.3

This test determines how efficiently you can move a large quantity of air out of the respiratory passageways. It also detects the existence of certain pulmonary diseases (e.g., asthma).

Instructions: To obtain a good recording, the following directions must be carried out quickly:

1. While the subject is breathing normal tidal volumes through the spirometer, have the subject inhale maximally (IRV).

2. Immediately turn the paper speed to maximum (20 mm/sec).

3. Give the subject a signal to exhale forcefully, smoothly, all the way by maximal expiration (ERV). After a good recording is obtained, remove the subject from the spirometer.

Data Analysis

1. Note the point where forced expiration first begins.

2. Draw a vertical line straight down past the point of expiration.

3. Draw a horizontal line from the point of maximal expiration until it intersects the vertical line.

4. On the horizontal line, make a mark every 20 mm and label each mark as a second (0, 1, 2, 3, etc.) (since the paper speed is 20 mm/sec, each 20 mm is 1 second).

5. At the 1-second mark, draw a line up until it intersects the falling pen mark. Mark this spot very clearly with an "X." This is the $FEV_{1.0}$.

6. To determine the volume of air expelled in the first second ($FEV_{1.0}$), measure how many centimeters the pen dropped from the top of the recording to the point of intersection.

Acid Test of Expired Air

1. Breathe through a straw into a solution containing the following:

   ■ 200 mL of water
   ■ 5 mL of 0.1 M NaOH
   ■ Three drops of phenolphthalein (color indicator for basic solution)

2. Record the number of seconds it takes to make the PURPLE solution turn CLEAR (like water).

   _____

   _____

3. Exercise vigorously for 3 minutes and repeat the earlier experiment. Are there any differences?

   _____

   _____

   _____

$$CO_2 + H_2O \underset{\xleftarrow{\hspace{3cm}}}{\xrightarrow{\text{Carbonic anhydrase}}} H_2CO_3 \underset{\xleftarrow{\hspace{2cm}}}{\xrightarrow{\hspace{2cm}}} H^+ + HCO_3^-$$

4. Use this equation to explain the differences you have observed.

   _____

   _____

   _____

   _____

Effects of Hyperventilation on Breath Holding

Exercise 12.5

1. While at rest, take a deep breath and hold it for as long as you can. Record this time in seconds.

   _____

2. Several minutes after regaining a normal breathing pattern, hyperventilate by breathing deeply at a rate of 18 to 22 times in a minute. Repeat the procedure given in step 1.

3. Record your results in the following table:

Student	Breath-holding Time	Breath-holding Time After Hyperventilation

4. Explain why you can hold your breath longer after hyperventilation.

   _____

   _____

   _____

   _____

The Respiratory Cycle

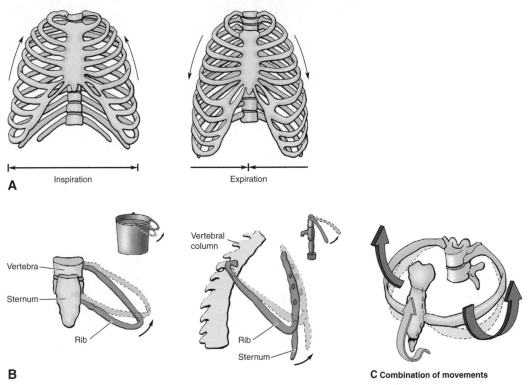

Figure 12.3 Muscles of respiration.

Study Questions

1. Which muscles are involved in breathing?

_____

_____

_____

_____

2. Describe how negative pressure is involved in breathing.

_____

_____

_____

_____

The Endocrine System

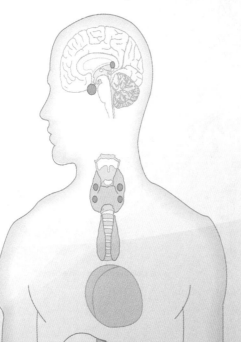
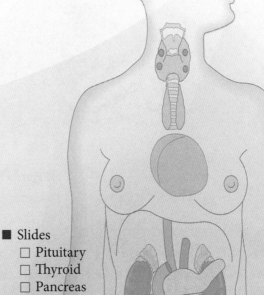

Objectives

After completing this laboratory exercise, students will be able to:

1. Name and identify the major organs of the endocrine system.
2. Identify specific histological specimens of endocrine tissue.
3. Identify the origin of specific hormones.
4. Describe the action of specific hormones on their target tissues.

Lab Materials

- Models of endocrine tissue (brain with pituitary gland, thyroid gland, pancreas, kidney with adrenal gland)
- Microscopes
- Slides
  - ☐ Pituitary
  - ☐ Thyroid
  - ☐ Pancreas

Exercises

Exercise 13.1: Organs and glands of the endocrine system

Exercise 13.2: The hypothalamus and the pituitary gland

    13.2-1: Hormones of the pituitary gland

Exercise 13.3: The thyroid gland

Exercise 13.4: The parathyroid glands

Exercise 13.5: The adrenal glands

Exercise 13.6: The pancreas

Estimated lab time: 60 minutes

Organs and Glands of the Endocrine System

The endocrine system is composed of several organs and glands. Figure 13.1 depicts the major endocrine tissues.

Instructions: Refer to your textbook as a guide to identify each tissue in the figure as well as on the models provided by your instructor.

- Adrenal gland
- Ovary
- Pancreas
- Parathyroid glands
- Pineal gland
- Pituitary gland
- Testis
- Thymus
- Thyroid gland

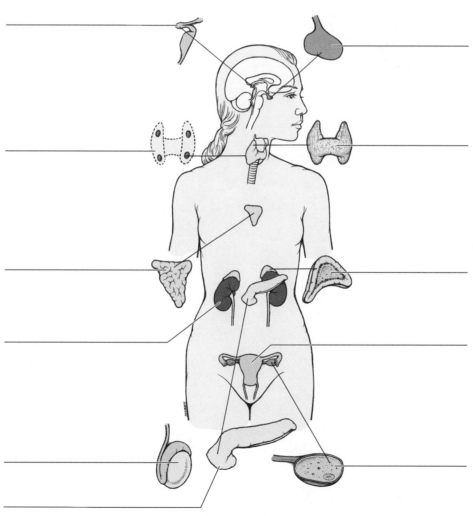

Figure 13.1

The Hypothalamus and the Pituitary Gland

Exercise 13.2

Instructions: Identify the following structures in Figure 13.2:

- Hypothalamus
- Adenohypophysis
- Neurohypophysis
- Infundibulum

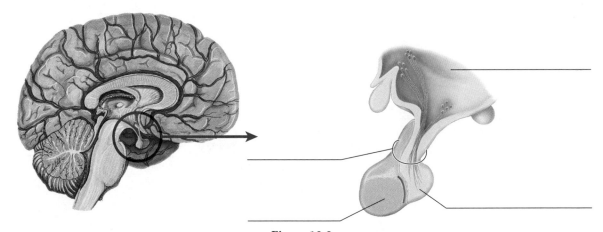

Figure 13.2

Instructions: Refer to your textbook as a guide to fill in the blanks in the following table to complete the name, action, or effect of the trophic or hormone-stimulating hormones of the hypothalamus:

Trophic Hormone	Inhibiting or Releasing	Effect
Thyrotropin-releasing hormone		Promotes secretion of thyroid-stimulating hormone
		Promotes secretion of adrenocorticotropic hormone
Gonadotropin-releasing hormone	Releasing	
Growth hormone–releasing hormone		Promotes secretion of growth hormone
	Inhibiting	Inhibits the secretion of prolactin

Hormones of the Pituitary Gland

Exercise 13.2-1

The pituitary gland is in fact composed of two glands, the anterior pituitary and the posterior pituitary. The hypothalamus stimulates both the anterior pituitary and the posterior pituitary to release specific hormones into circulation.

Instructions: In Figure 13.3, indicate the hormone released that would affect the target tissue shown.

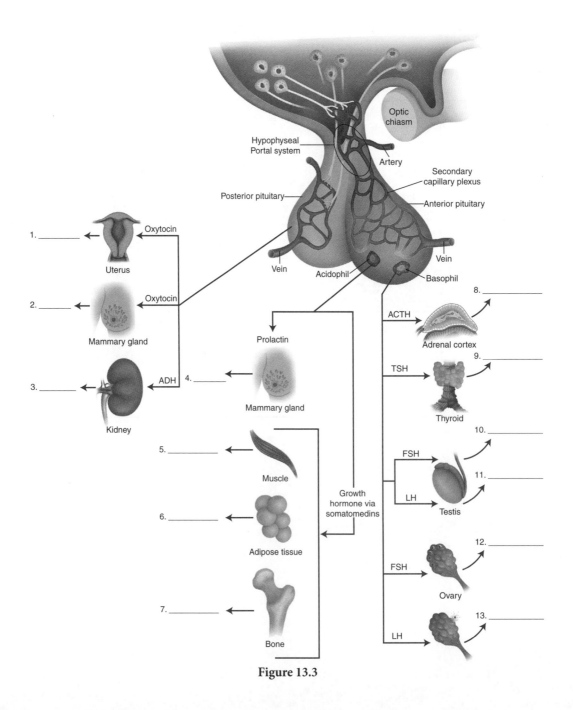

Figure 13.3

Hormones of the Posterior Pituitary Gland

Instructions: Refer to your textbook to complete the following table:

Hormone	Action
Antidiuretic hormone	
Oxytocin	

Hormones of the Anterior Pituitary Gland

Instructions: Refer to your textbook to complete the following table:

Hormone	Action
Follicle-stimulating hormone	Female: Male:
Luteinizing hormone	Female: Male:
Thyroid-stimulating hormone	
Adrenocorticotropic hormone	
Prolactin	Female: Male:
Growth hormone	

The Thyroid Gland

Instructions: Identify the following structures in Figure 13.4:

- Thyroid cartilage
- Thyroid gland
- Trachea

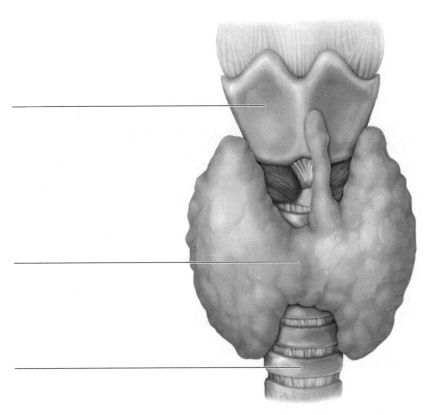

Figure 13.4

Instructions: In the micrograph (Figure 13.5), identify the large colloid. What is the colloid and what is its purpose and function?

_____

_____

_____

_____

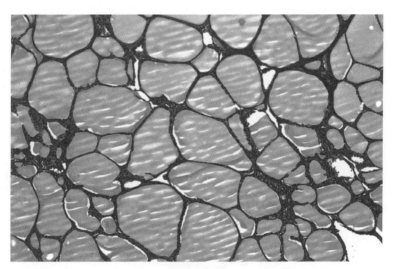

Figure 13.5

Hormones of the Thyroid Gland

Instructions: Refer to your textbook to complete the following table:

Cell Type	Hormone	Target	Action
Follicular cells	T3 and T4 (thyroxine)		Increases metabolism in all cells
		Osteoclasts	Inhibits osteoclasts and works to reduce calcium levels in the blood

Exercise 13.4   The Parathyroid Glands

Instructions: Identify the following structures in Figure 13.6:

- All the parathyroid glands
- Thyroid gland
- Trachea

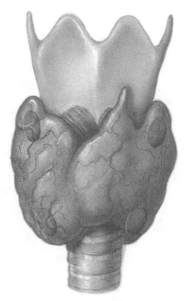

Figure 13.6

Study Questions

1. Are the parathyroid glands located on the anterior or posterior surface of the thyroid gland?

    _____

    _____

    _____

2. Which hormone is released from the chief cells of the parathyroid gland? Which organ(s) is its target? What is its action?

    _____

    _____

    _____

The Adrenal Glands

Instructions: Identify the following structures in Figure 13.7 (terms may be used more than once):

1. Adrenal cortex

- Zona glomerulosa
- Zona fasciculate
- Zona reticularis

2. Adrenal medulla

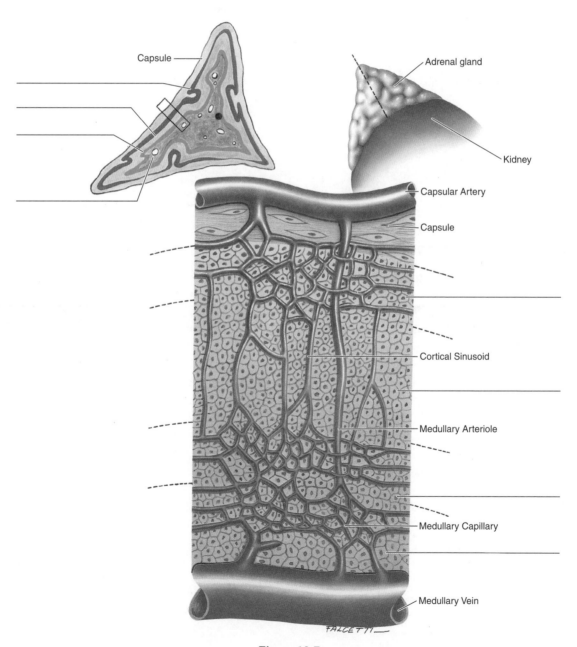

Figure 13.7

Hormones of the Adrenal Cortex

Instructions: Refer to your textbook to complete the following table:

Zone	Hormone	Target	Action
Zona glomerulosa	Aldosterone		Stimulates sodium _____ Stimulates potassium _____
	Cortisol	Most cells of the body	Stimulates _____ from the catabolism of proteins and fats
Zona reticularis		Most cells of the body	

Hormones of the Adrenal Medulla

Instructions: Refer to your textbook to complete the following table:

Zone	Hormone	Target	Action
Adrenal medulla (chromaffin cells)		Many cell types	

The Pancreas

Instructions: Identify the following structures in Figure 13.8:

- Tail of pancreas
- Pancreatic ducts (note if they endocrine or exocrine)
- Bile duct
- Head of pancreas
- Islets of Langerhans

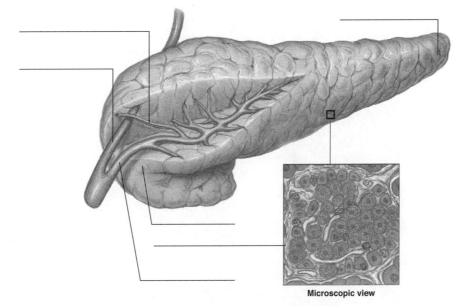

Microscopic view

Figure 13.8

Hormones of the Pancreatic Islet

There are several cell types found in the pancreatic islet.

Instructions: Refer to your textbook to complete the following table:

Cell Type	Hormone	Target	Action
Alpha cells		Liver and adipose tissue	Elevates blood glucose level
	Insulin		Stimulates glucose entry into cells and acts to reduce blood glucose level

The Digestive System

Objectives

After completing this laboratory exercise, students will be able to:

1. Describe the basic anatomy of the gastrointestinal tract.
2. Describe the gross and microscopic anatomy of specific regions of the gastrointestinal tract.

Overview

This lab exercise is designed to familiarize you with the basic anatomy of the digestive tract. Examine each organ and tissue in order as you progress through the gastrointestinal tract from the mouth to the anus.

Lab Materials

- Models of the following organs and structures:
  - ☐ The oral cavity
  - ☐ Stomach
  - ☐ Small intestine
  - ☐ Large intestine
  - ☑ Liver/gallbladder
  - ☐ Pancreas
- Histological preparations of the following tissues:
  - ☐ Liver
  - ☐ Pancreas

Exercises

Exercise 14.1: The oral cavity and the pharynx
Exercise 14.2: The esophagus
Exercise 14.3: The stomach
Exercise 14.4: The small intestine
Exercise 14.5: The large intestine
Exercise 14.6: The liver and the gallbladder
Exercise 14.7: The pancreas

Estimated lab time: 90 minutes

The Oral Cavity and the Pharynx

Instructions: Refer to your textbook to find and label the following structures in Figure 14.1 and on the model:

- Teeth
- Hard palate
- Soft palate
- Tongue
- Epiglottis
- Pharynx
- Esophagus
- Submandibular gland
- Parotid gland
- Sublingual gland

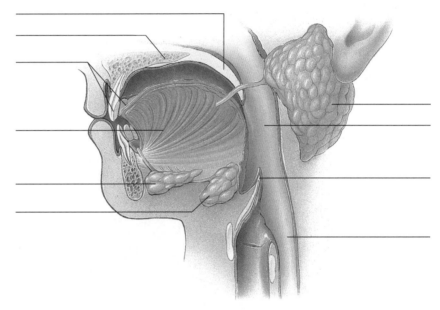

Figure 14.1

Study Questions

1. What is mastication?

_____

_____

_____

2. How do the teeth and tongue work together?

_____

_____

_____

3. Which enzyme is present in saliva that begins the digestion of starch?

_____

_____

_____

Exercise 14.2

The Esophagus

Instructions: Refer to your textbook to find and label the following structures in Figure 14.2 and on the models:

- Tongue
- Oropharynx
- Esophagus (use twice)
- Liver
- Gallbladder
- Stomach (use twice)
- Diaphragm

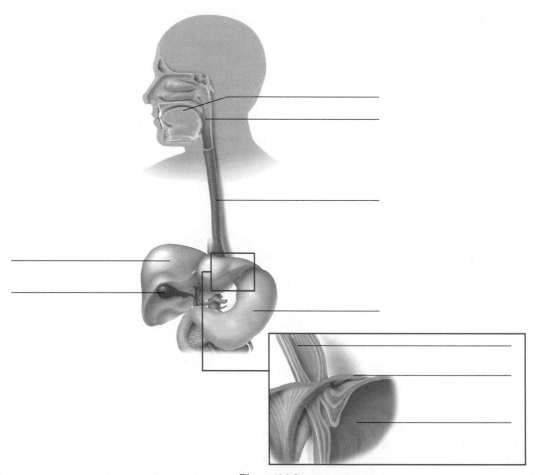

Figure 14.2

Study Questions

1. What type of muscular contraction occurs in the esophagus?

_____

_____

_____

2. What is the function of the mucosal layer?

_____

_____

_____

3. What happens if the lower esophageal sphincter is weak?

_____

_____

_____

The Stomach

Exercise 14.3

Instructions: Refer to your textbook to find and label the following structures in Figure 14.3 and on the models:

- Longitudinal layer of smooth muscle
- Circular layer of smooth muscle
- Oblique layer of smooth muscle
- Mucosa
- Esophagus
- Fundus
- Cardiac region
- Body
- Greater and lesser curvature
- Pyloric region

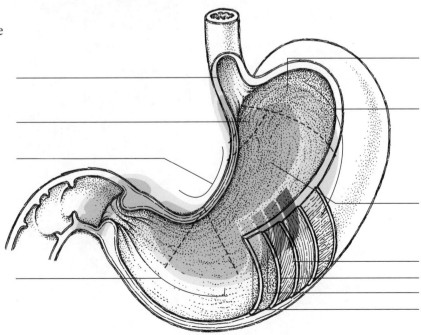

Figure 14.3

Study Questions

1. Which enzyme is released in the stomach? Upon activation, what nutrient does it digest?

_____

_____

_____

2. What prevents the digestive juices from damaging the stomach?

_____

_____

_____

Exercise 14.4	The Small Intestine

Instructions: Refer to your textbook to find and label the following structures in Figure 14.4 and on the models:

- Jejunum
- Duodenum
- Ileum
- Cecum
- Appendix

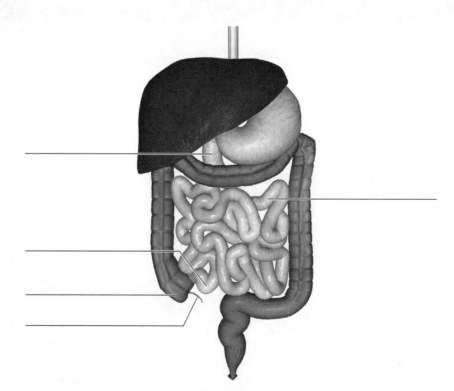

Figure 14.4

Study Questions

1. Propose a possible reason for the changes in epithelia in the three regions of the small intestine.

   _____

   _____

   _____

2. What is the principal function of the small intestine?

   _____

   _____

   _____

3. Which ducts carry secretions from the liver and pancreas into the duodenum?

   _____

   _____

   _____

The Large Intestine

Instructions: Refer to your textbook to find and label the following structures in Figure 14.5 and on the models:

- Ascending colon
- Transverse colon
- Descending colon
- Rectum
- Greater omentum

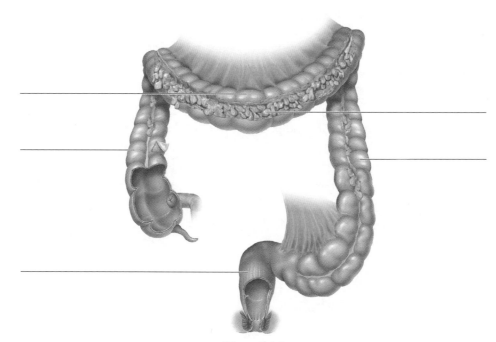

Figure 14.5

Study Questions

1. Describe the role of the large intestine in the digestive process.

_____

_____

_____

2. Observe the microscopic slide of colon epithelium. What type of cells are present and why?

_____

_____

_____

The Liver and the Gallbladder

Instructions: Refer to your textbook to find and label the following structures in Figure 14.6 and on the models:

- ◾ Left lobe of liver
- ◾ Right lobe of liver
- ◾ Gallbladder

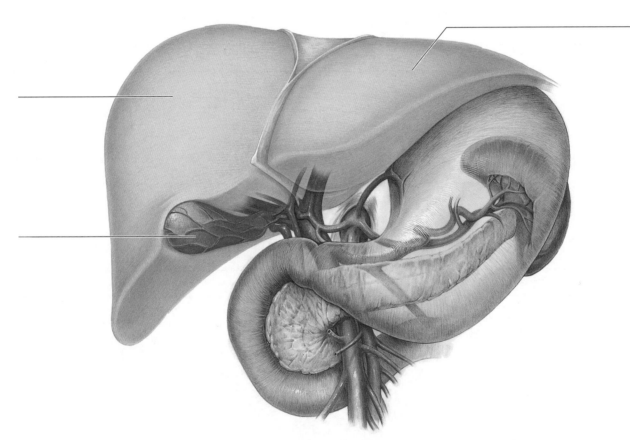

Figure 14.6

Study Questions

1. Describe the location of the gallbladder in relation to the liver.

   _____

   _____

   _____

2. Discuss the function of the gallbladder.

   _____

   _____

   _____

3. What is the general term for cells that compose the liver?

   _____

   _____

   _____

4. List the functions of the liver.

   _____

   _____

   _____

The Pancreas

Instructions: Refer to your textbook to find and label the following structures in Figure 14.7 and on the models:

- Common bile duct
- Pancreatic duct
- Alpha cells
- Beta cells
- Delta cells

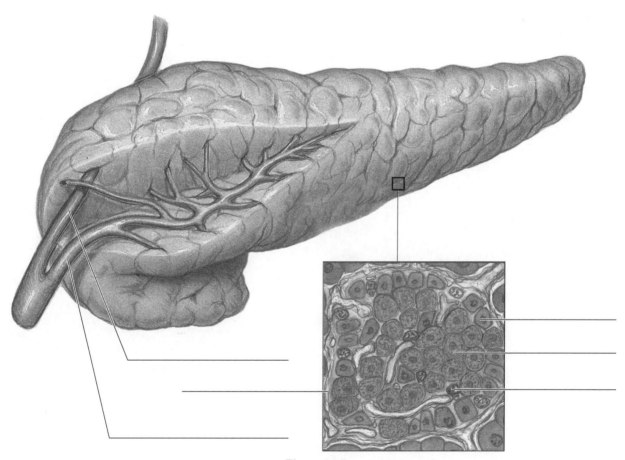

Figure 14.7

Study Questions

1. Discuss why the pancreas is both an exocrine and an endocrine gland.

   _____

   _____

   _____

2. Discuss the route by which pancreatic juices flow into the duodenum.

   _____

   _____

   _____

3. Discuss the role of the pancreas in the digestive process.

   _____

   _____

   _____

The Urinary System

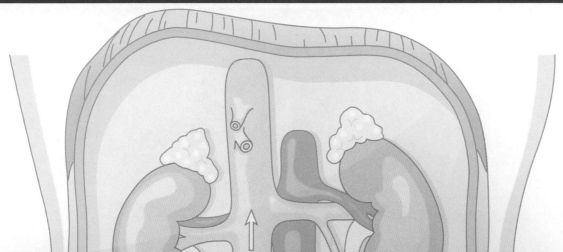

Objectives

After completing this laboratory exercise, students will be able to:

1. Identify the anatomic components of the urinary system.
2. Identify the anatomic structures of the kidney.
3. Describe the structure of the nephron and the basic aspects of urine formation.
4. Describe the histological structures of the urinary system.

Overview

The urinary system includes the kidneys, bladder, ureters, and urethra. These organs and tissues control the amount of water and salts that are absorbed back into the blood and what is secreted as waste as a result of filtering the blood. This lab exercise is designed to introduce you to the major organs and structures of the urinary tract as well as the production of urine.

Lab Materials

■ Models of the following organs and structures:
  ☐ Kidney
  ☐ Bladder
  ☐ Urinary tract
■ Histological preparations of the following tissues:
  ☐ Glomerulus
  ☐ Transitional epithelium of the bladder
■ Preserved sheep kidney

Exercises

Exercise 15.1: Urinary anatomy
Exercise 15.2: The anatomic structure of the kidney
Exercise 15.3: The functional unit of the kidney, the nephron
Exercise 15.4: The glomerulus
Exercise 15.5: The bladder
Exercise 15.6: Characteristics of normal urine

Estimated lab time: 90 minutes

Exercise 15.1

Urinary Anatomy

Instructions: In Figure 15.1, label the following structures of the urinary system:

- Kidneys
- Ureters
- Bladder
- Urethra

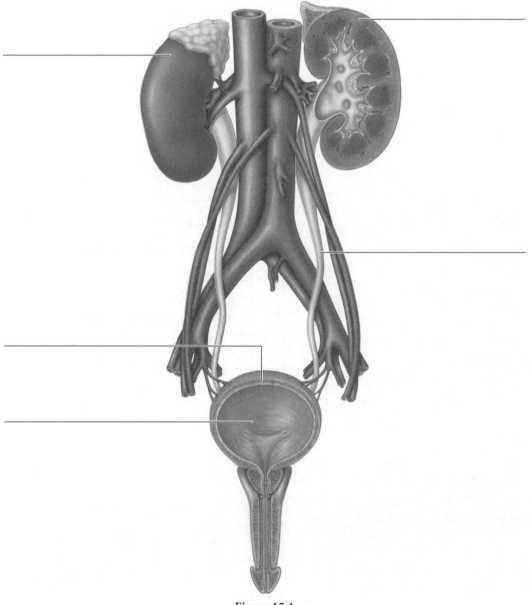

Figure 15.1

Instructions: Explain the function of each of the following structures:

1. Kidneys:

_____

_____

_____

2. Ureters:

_____

_____

_____

3. Bladder:

_____

_____

_____

4. Urethra:

_____

_____

_____

The Anatomic Structure of the Kidney

Instructions: Obtain a sheep kidney from your instructor or a model of the human kidney. Observe a coronal cut through the kidney and label the following structures in Figure 15.2. Locate as many structures as possible on the kidney model.

■ Hilum
■ Cortex
■ Pyramid
■ Major calyx
■ Minor calyx
■ Renal pelvis
■ Ureter
■ Abdominal aorta
■ Inferior vena cava
■ Renal artery
■ Renal vein

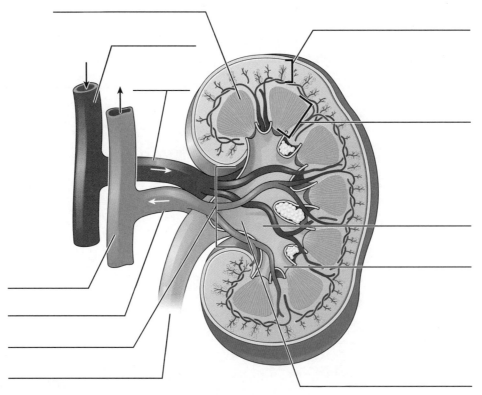

Figure 15.2

The Functional Unit of the Kidney, the Nephron

Instructions: Locate the following structures in Figure 15.3

- Ascending limb of loop of Henle
- Bowman's capsule
- Descending limb of loop of Henle
- Distal convoluted tubule

- Glomerulus
- Proximal convoluted tubule
- Renal corpuscle

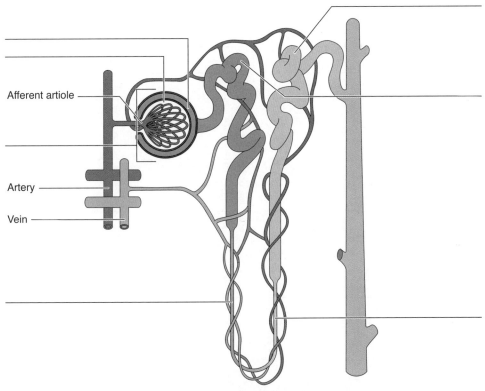

Afferent artiole

Artery

Vein

Figure 15.3

Instructions: Now explain the physiological action that occurs at each point.

1. Renal corpuscle:

_____

_____

_____

2. Bowman's capsule:

_____

_____

_____

3. Glomerulus:

_____

_____

_____

4. Proximal convoluted tubule:

_____

_____

_____

5. Descending limb of loop of Henle:

_____

_____

_____

6. Ascending limb of loop of Henle:

_____

_____

_____

7. Distal convoluted tubule:

_____

_____

_____

Study Question

What type of cells line the nephron?

_____

_____

The Glomerulus

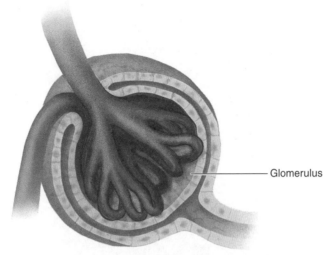

Glomerulus

Figure 15.4

Instructions:

1. Observe and describe the glomerulus section on the microscope.

_____

_____

_____

_____

_____

2. Explain how the glomerulus filters the blood. What are the three layers of the filtration membrane?

_____

_____

_____

_____

_____

Exercise 15.5   The Bladder

Instructions: Label the following structures in Figure 15.5:

- Detrusor
- Ureteric openings
- Urinary trigone
- Internal urethral sphincter
- Urethra

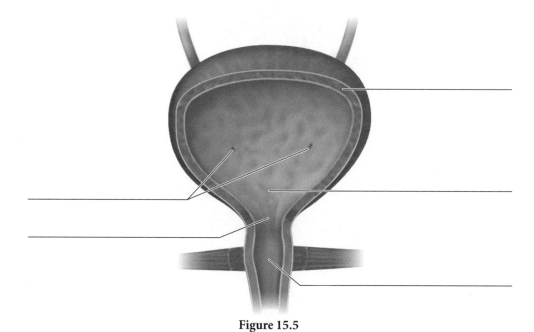

Figure 15.5

Instructions: Observe the slide of transitional epithelium. What is the functional significance of transitional epithelium?

_____

_____

_____

Characteristics of Normal Urine

Characteristic	Normal
pH	4.5–8
Specific gravity	1.003–1.03
Water content	93–97%
Volume	1200 mL/day
Color	Clear yellow
Odor	Variable with composition
Bacterial content	Sterile

Urine is much easier to assess than blood and provides a window to renal and cardiovascular function. The table shows the normal characteristics of urine.

Instructions: Using what you have learned about renal function and what is given in the table, answer the following questions regarding abnormal urinary readings:

Study Questions

1. Your patient has white blood cells in her urine. What is the possible cause?

   _____

   _____

   _____

2. Your patient has a urinary pH of 8.5. What is the possible cause?

   _____

   _____

   _____

3. Your patient has a urinary volume of 400 mL/day. What might be happening?

   _____

   _____

   _____

The Male and Female Reproductive Systems

Objectives

After completing this laboratory exercise, students will be able to:

1. Name the major organs of the male and female reproductive tract.
2. Identify the major organs and tissues of the male and female reproductive tract.
3. Identify and name the tissues and structures of the breast that are associated with lactation.
4. Describe the basic functions of organs and tissues of the male and female reproductive tract.

Overview

The male and female reproductive systems produce sperm and egg (the gametes) that merge to form a developing fetus. In this laboratory exercise, you will become familiar with the tissues and organs of each system and understand both systems' basic anatomy and physiology.

Lab Materials

Models of the following organs and structures:

- Male reproductive system
- Testicle
- Female reproductive system
- Uterus
- Histological preparations of the following tissue:
  - ☐ Ovary
  - ☐ Corpus luteum
  - ☐ Primary follicle
  - ☐ Secondary follicle

Exercises

Exercise 16.1: Male reproductive anatomy

Exercise 16.2: Male reproductive anatomy: The testis

Exercise 16.3: Female reproductive anatomy

Exercise 16.4: Female reproductive anatomy: Structure of the ovary

Exercise 16.5: Female reproductive anatomy: The breast

Estimated lab time: 90 minutes

Male Reproductive Anatomy

Instructions: Locate and identify the following structures in Figure 16.1 and on the models:

- Urinary bladder
- Pubic symphysis
- Ductus (vas) deferens
- Shaft of penis
- Corpus cavernosum
- Corpus spongiosum
- Epididymis
- Glans penis
- Testis
- Scrotum
- Ampulla of ductus deferens
- Prostate gland
- Bulbourethral gland
- Urethra
- Ureter
- Seminal vesicle
- Ejaculatory duct

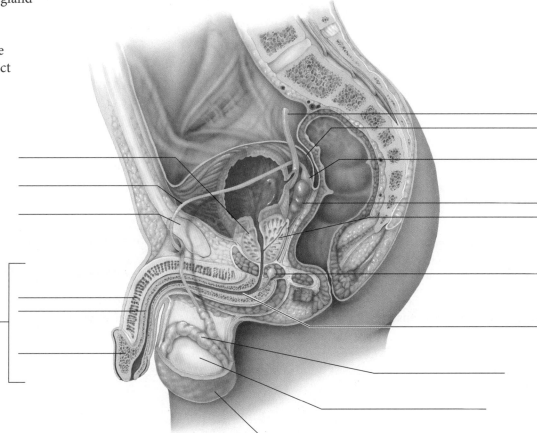

Figure 16.1

Instructions: Locate and identify the following structures in Figure 16.2 and find them on the models:

- Urinary bladder
- Corpus cavernosum
- Corpus spongiosum
- Bulb of penis
- Crus of penis
- Glans penis
- Prostate gland
- Bulbourethral gland
- Urethra

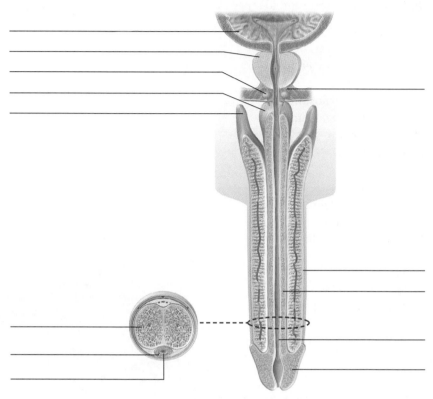

Figure 16.2

Study Questions

1. Which structures constitute the external anatomy of the male reproductive system?

   _____

   _____

   _____

2. What is the function of the cremaster muscle?

   _____

   _____

   _____

Male Reproductive Anatomy: The Testis

Exercise 16.2

Instructions: Locate and identify the following structures in Figure 16.3 and find them on the models:

- Epididymis
- Ductus (vas) deferens
- Cremaster
- Efferent ductule
- Seminiferous tubule
- Lobule of epididymis
- Tunica vaginalis
- Spermatic cord

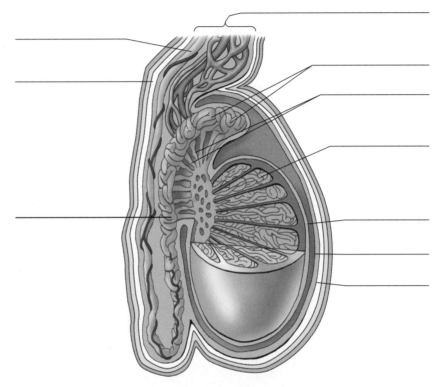

Figure 16.3

Study Questions

1. How is the testis maintained at a temperature lower than body temperature?

_____

_____

_____

2. What is the function of the prostate?

_____

_____

_____

| Exercise 16.3 | Female Reproductive Anatomy |

Instructions: Locate and identify the following structures in Figure 16.4 and find them on the models:

- Uterine tube
- Ovary
- Posterior fornix
- Cervix
- Vagina
- Uterus
- Urinary bladder
- Pubic symphysis
- Urethra
- Clitoris
- Labium minus
- Labium majus

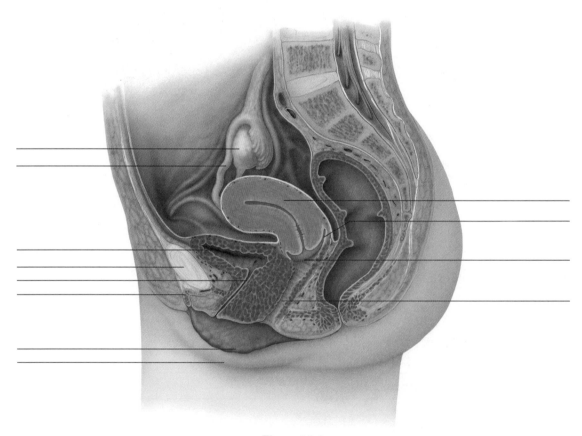

Figure 16.4

Instructions: Locate and identify the following structures in Figure 16.5 and find them on the models:

- Fimbria
- Ovary
- Myometrium
- Endometrium
- Cervical canal
- Cervix
- Vagina
- Uterine tube
- Fundus
- Body

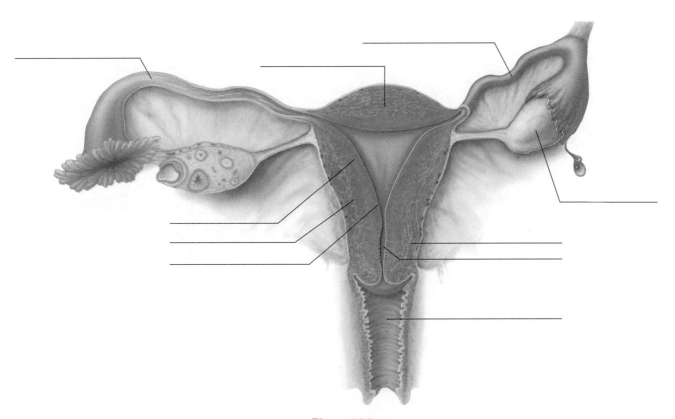

Figure 16.5

Female Reproductive Anatomy: Structure of the Ovary

Instructions: Locate and identify the following structures in Figure 16.6 and find them on the models:

- Medulla
- Cortex
- Corpus luteum
- Fimbria

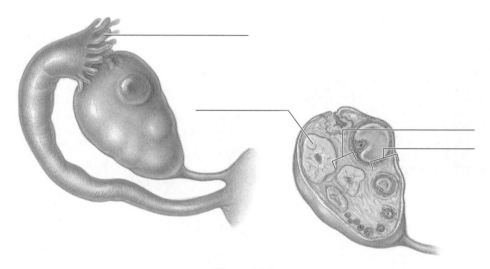

Figure 16.6

Female Reproductive Anatomy: The Breast

Exercise 16.5

Instructions: Locate and identify the following structures in Figure 16.7 and find them on the models:

- Suspensory ligament
- Lobules
- Adipose tissue

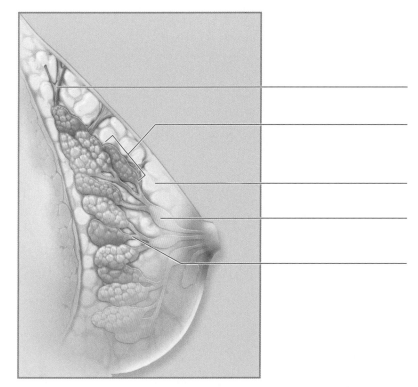

Figure 16.7

Study Questions

1. What are myoepithelial cells and what is their function?

_____

_____

_____

2. What is the function of the suspensory ligament?

_____

_____

_____